In Silico approach towards magnetic fluid hyperthermia of cancer treatment

In Silico approach towards magnetic fluid hyperthermia of cancer treatment

Modeling and simulation

Muhammad Suleman
Department of Mathematics, Riphah Institute of Computing and Applied Sciences (RICAS), Riphah International University, Lahore, Pakistan

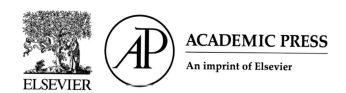

Academic Press is an imprint of Elsevier
125 London Wall, London EC2Y 5AS, United Kingdom
525 B Street, Suite 1650, San Diego, CA 92101, United States
50 Hampshire Street, 5th Floor, Cambridge, MA 02139, United States
The Boulevard, Langford Lane, Kidlington, Oxford OX5 1GB, United Kingdom

Copyright © 2023 Elsevier Inc. All rights reserved.

No part of this publication may be reproduced or transmitted in any form or by any means, electronic or mechanical, including photocopying, recording, or any information storage and retrieval system, without permission in writing from the publisher. Details on how to seek permission, further information about the Publisher's permissions policies and our arrangements with organizations such as the Copyright Clearance Center and the Copyright Licensing Agency, can be found at our website: www.elsevier.com/permissions.

This book and the individual contributions contained in it are protected under copyright by the Publisher (other than as may be noted herein).

Notices
Knowledge and best practice in this field are constantly changing. As new research and experience broaden our understanding, changes in research methods, professional practices, or medical treatment may become necessary.

Practitioners and researchers must always rely on their own experience and knowledge in evaluating and using any information, methods, compounds, or experiments described herein. In using such information or methods they should be mindful of their own safety and the safety of others, including parties for whom they have a professional responsibility.

To the fullest extent of the law, neither the Publisher nor the authors, contributors, or editors, assume any liability for any injury and/or damage to persons or property as a matter of products liability, negligence or otherwise, or from any use or operation of any methods, products, instructions, or ideas contained in the material herein.

ISBN 978-0-443-13286-5

For information on all Academic Press publications
visit our website at https://www.elsevier.com/books-and-journals

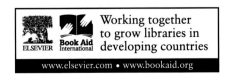

Publisher: Stacy Masucci
Acquisitions Editor: Linda Versteeg-Buschman
Editorial Project Manager: Sam Young
Production Project Manager: Sajana Devasi P K
Cover Designer: Christian J. Bilbow

Typeset by STRAIVE, India

Contents

Introduction .... *xi*

Chapter 1: Basics of magnetic fluid hyperthermia 1
   1.1 What is nanoscience and nanotechnology? 1
   1.2 Basic types of biological experiments 1
       1.2.1 The in vitro studies 1
       1.2.2 The in vivo studies 2
       1.2.3 The in silico studies 2
   1.3 Fundamental types of cancer and its statistics 2
   1.4 Traditional techniques used for cancer treatment 2
       1.4.1 Chemotherapy 3
       1.4.2 Radiotherapy 3
       1.4.3 Surgery 3
       1.4.4 Immunotherapy 3
   1.5 Hyperthermia 4
   1.6 Major types of hyperthermia 4
       1.6.1 Moderate or mild hyperthermia 5
       1.6.2 Ablation hyperthermia 5
       1.6.3 Diathermia 5
       1.6.4 Local hyperthermia 6
       1.6.5 Regional hyperthermia 6
       1.6.6 Whole-body hyperthermia 6
       1.6.7 Interstitial hyperthermia 6
   1.7 Magnetic nanoparticles (MNPs) and hyperthermia 6
   1.8 Synthesis of MNPs 7
       1.8.1 Synthesis of $CoFe_2O_4@MnFe_2O_4$ MNPs through modification of growth method 8
       1.8.2 Synthesis of Fe_3O_4 MNPs by the method of Molday 8
       1.8.3 Synthesis of Fe_3O_4 MNPs by facile method 9
   1.9 Loading MNPs at the tumor site 10
       1.9.1 Intravenous injection approach 10
       1.9.2 Direct needle injection approach 10
   1.10 Types of flow 11
       1.10.1 Steady and unsteady flow 11
       1.10.2 Uniform and nonuniform flow 12

Contents

    1.10.3 Laminar and turbulent flow 12
    1.10.4 Compressible and incompressible flow 12
    1.10.5 Rotational and irrotational flows 12
    1.10.6 One-, two-, and three-dimensional flow 12
  1.11 Blood vessels 12
    1.11.1 Arteries 13
    1.11.2 Veins 13
    1.11.3 Capillaries 13
  References 13

Chapter 2: Historical background of magnetic fluid hyperthermia 17
  2.1 Mathematical modeling approach toward MFH 17
  2.2 Analytical modeling of MFH 25
  2.3 Numerical modeling of MFH 25
  2.4 Optimization in MFH 26
  2.5 Integrated therapies 27
  2.6 In vivo experimental studies of MFH 28
  2.7 In vitro experimental studies on MFH 29
  2.8 Case study on MFH 29
  References 30

Chapter 3: The phenomena of heat dissipation by magnetic nanoparticles under applied magnetic field 37
  3.1 The force acting on nanoparticles under an applied magnetic field 37
  3.2 Maxwell's equations of electromagnetism 37
  3.3 The magnetic vector potential 38
  3.4 The scalar electric potential 38
  3.5 Hysteresis curve and coercivity 39
  3.6 Neel and Brownian relaxation 39
  3.7 Heat dissipation by MNPs 41
  3.8 Different heating sources used in magnetic fluid hyperthermia 43
    3.8.1 Radio frequency heating 44
    3.8.2 Microwave heating 44
    3.8.3 Ultrasound heating 44
    3.8.4 Infrared radiation heating 44
    3.8.5 Laser heating 44
  References 44

Chapter 4: Mathematical models of physical processes involved in magnetic fluid hyperthermia 47
  4.1 Modeling nanofluid flow in the injecting needle 47
  4.2 Modeling nanofluid infusion in the tumor interstitium 47
  4.3 Modeling nanofluid diffusion in the tumor interstitium 48
  4.4 Modeling transfer of heat in the body tissue 48
  4.5 Modeling estimation of a fraction of tumor injury 49

4.6 Physical properties of the nanofluid 49
    4.6.1 The volume fraction of the nanofluid 49
    4.6.2 Effective density of the nanofluid 50
    4.6.3 Nanofluid's specific heat capacity 50
    4.6.4 Nanofluid's thermal conductivity 50
    4.6.5 The viscosity of the nanofluid 50
4.7 Flux of the nanofluid 50
4.8 Nanofluid's mass concentration 51
4.9 Boundary conditions (BCs) 51
    4.9.1 Neumann boundary condition 51
    4.9.2 Dirichlet boundary condition 51
4.10 Initial conditions (ICs) 52
References 52

Chapter 5: Mathematical modeling and simulation of magnetic fluid hyperthermia of liver tumor 53

5.1 Mathematical modeling formulation of the problem 55
    5.1.1 Nanofluid injection in the tumor 55
    5.1.2 Nanofluid diffusion in the tumor 56
    5.1.3 Heat dissipation by the MNPs 56
    5.1.4 Transfer of heat in the liver tumor tissue 57
    5.1.5 Estimation of the fraction of tissue necrosis 57
    5.1.6 Heat sources in terms of concentration and temperature 58
5.2 Results 59
5.3 Conclusions 70
References 71

Chapter 6: Modeling thermal therapy of poroelastic brain tumor using magnetic nanoparticles 73

6.1 Problem statement and strategy to handle the problem 75
6.2 Deformation of poroelastic tumor 77
6.3 Transport of the nanofluid in poroelastic tumor 78
6.4 Heat produced by the MNPs in the poroelastic brain tissue 79
6.5 Heat transfer in poroelastic brain tissue 80
6.6 The degree of tumor injury 80
6.7 Implementation in COMSOL multiphysics 81
6.8 Results and discussions 82
6.9 Conclusions 92
References 93

Chapter 7: Finite element modeling analysis of hyperthermia of female breast cancer in three dimensions 95

7.1 Physical properties of nanofluid 96
7.2 Mathematical modeling formulation of the problem 96

Contents

    7.2.1 Nanofluid infusion in the tumor..96
    7.2.2 The diffusion of nanofluid in the tumor 97
    7.2.3 Heat produced by Fe_3O_4 MNPs 97
    7.2.4 Heat transfer in the breast tissue..98
    7.2.5 Prediction of the fraction of tumor necrosis 98
7.3 Sensitivity analysis 98
7.4 The AMF generated by the coil 99
7.5 Results...99
7.6 Conclusions...112
References...112

Chapter 8: Mathematical modeling and simulation of enhanced permeation and retention (EPR) effect with thermal analysis.. 115

8.1 Physical properties of nanofluid...116
8.2 Mathematical modeling formulation of the problem..117
    8.2.1 Nanofluid flow in the blood vessel 117
    8.2.2 Diffusion of nanoflow in the tumor interstitium 118
    8.2.3 Heat transfer in the porous tumor interstitium 118
8.3 Results and discussions 119
8.4 Conclusions...125
References...125

Chapter 9: Simulating the nanoflow around Happel's sphere in the porous tumor carrying the cell-model structure.. 127

9.1 Physical properties of nanofluids..128
9.2 Mathematical modeling formulation of the problem..128
    9.2.1 Nanofluid flow in the porous tumor 128
    9.2.2 Nanofluid diffusion in the tumor interstitium...128
9.3 Results...129
9.4 Conclusions...138
References...138

Chapter 10: Computational analysis of the reacting nanofluid in the porous tumor 139

10.1 Properties of nanofluid 139
10.2 Mathematical modeling formulation of the problem..139
10.3 Adding physics and geometry construction of the problem...................................141
10.4 Adding initial condition, boundary conditions, and material.................................142
10.5 Mesh generation of the problem 144
10.6 Results and discussions 144
10.7 Conclusions...148
References...149

Chapter 11: Thermal therapy of cylindrical tumor with optimization using Nelder-Mead method *151*

   11.1 Materials and methods 151
   11.2 Nanofluid and its properties 151
   11.3 Mathematical modeling formulation of the problem 152
        11.3.1 Magnetic flux density developed by a multiturn coil 152
        11.3.2 Steady-state analysis of bioheat transfer in liver tissue 152
        11.3.3 Analytical solution of steady-state bioheat transfer model 153
        11.3.4 Transient analytical of bioheat transfer in liver tissue 154
        11.3.5 Construction of optimization problem model 154
        11.3.6 Adding physics, studies, and geometry construction of the problem 154
        11.3.7 Adding a material, initial condition, and boundary conditions 155
        11.3.8 Mesh generation of the model 156
   11.4 Results 158
   11.5 Conclusions 162
   References 163

Supplementary material: Appendix A *165*
Supplementary material: Appendix B *167*
Supplementary material: Appendix C *169*
Supplementary material: Appendix D *173*
Supplementary material: Appendix E *177*
Conclusions *183*
Future work *187*
Index *189*

Introduction

Nanotechnology has the potential to present a more targeted approach to provide effective treatment improvements for cancer patients. Different research groups have demonstrated that magnetic nanoparticles (MNPs) can destroy cancer cells. The world has shown considerable interest in using nanomaterials for drug delivery and cancer therapy. Currently, radiotherapy, chemotherapy, surgery, and immunotherapy have been used as cancer treatment modalities, but these traditional treatment techniques have some drawbacks. Chemotherapy uses drugs to damage cancer cells, and it kills cancerous tissue along with the surrounding normal cells of the body as well. In radiotherapy, radiation is used to destroy the tumor. However, due to the difficulty in targeting the whole tumor, radiotherapy has destructive effects on the organs surrounding the tumor. Surgery is also inappropriate for deep-sited tumors, and immunotherapy fails if the immune system is not boosted enough to fight against cancer. Due to these drawbacks, scientists have researched alternative therapeutic tools. MNP-induced intracellular hyperthermia or magnetic fluid hyperthermia (MFH) is the therapeutic modality that has the ability to overcome these drawbacks.

MFH has been subjected to mathematical modeling and a simulation approach, contrary to costly and time-consuming in vivo and in vitro studies. In this research, the two types of MNPs, core-shell $CoFe_2O_4$@$MnFe_2O_4$ and Fe_3O_4 MNPs, being more biocompatible and the best for heat generation, have been employed. This book focuses on hyperthermia of liver, brain, and breast tumors. The finite element method (FEM)-based models of all hyperthermia processes involved in this treatment modality have been simulated and analyzed. The underlying mechanism involved in this therapy has been simulated. We have applied optimization techniques based on the Nelder Mead method to optimize the parameters involved in the therapy. In this therapeutic technique, MNPs are injected into the tumor. After MNPS are infused into the tumor, an external magnetic field is applied to heat the MNPs. Due to the Neel and Brownian relaxation effects, heat is released by the MNPs, which elevates the temperature of the tumor. The temperature of the tumor is raised to 45°C from the normal tissue temperature of 37°C. This heat is sufficient to produce hyperthermia, where the elevated temperature is maintained for a specified time in the tumor to destroy the tumor cells under heat stress.

In this book, we first review the mathematical modeling approach toward this treatment modality. A comprehensive literature survey of the physical process and models involved in this therapy is conducted. We review the MNPs that are applicable in MFH, the models involved in heat dissipation, the main factors affecting the heating efficiency, the

Introduction

thermophysical properties of nanofluid, and the in vitro and in vivo studies. The mathematical models involved in MFH are surveyed, including analytical solutions, numerical modeling, and major optimization techniques. The integration of hyperthermia with radiotherapy, chemotherapy, laser therapy, and immunotherapy is briefly discussed. The major challenges and opportunities facing MFH are also discussed.

Second, in silico study of MFH for the treatment of liver cancer using core-shell $CoFe_2O_4$@$MnFe_2O_4$ MNPs because exchange coupling between a magnetically hardcore and a magnetically softshell can enhance the properties of MNPs to maximize the power loss generated by them. The hyperthermia process includes: (1) nanofluid infusion is modeled by pressure-driven Darcy's Law coupled with the simple mass conservation principle, (2) nanofluid diffusion in the tumor is modeled by the convection-diffusion equation, (3) after diffusion, the MNPs are activated with the application of an applied magnetic field (AMF) that produces heat released by vibrating MNPs following Brownian and Neel relaxation effects, (4) the dissipated heat is transferred in the tissue following Penne's bioheat transfer model (PBHTM), (5) at elevated temperature, tumor cells are damaged, and (6) the fraction of the tumor cells damaged is predicted using the Arrhenius kinetic model. The transfer of heat in liver tissue and tumor thermal damage are subject to ICs and BCs, based on FEM-based model analysis. All these processes are simulated using COMSOL Multiphysics software to predict the pressure, velocity, concentration, temperature distribution, and the fraction of tumor damage during treatment. The expressions for temperature and concentration-dependent heat sources are derived and compared with a constant source of heat. Simulations show that the concentration-dependent source of heat produced a higher temperature compared to the remaining two heat sources.

Third, the Fe_3O_4 MNPs in the in silico study for the hyperthermia treatment of the poroelastic brain tumor have been incorporated. The deformation of the brain tissue based on a stress-and-strain relationship is simulated and analyzed using FEM numerical models on COMSOL Multiphysics along with other hyperthermia processes. The validation of the simulations with the preexisting experimental studies advocates successful thermal therapy of the brain tumor.

Fourth, a three-dimensional (3D) simulation study to treat breast tumors using Fe_3O_4 MNPs is performed. The hyperthermia process is simulated on COMSOL Multiphysics using 3D FEM models of corresponding phenomena. The backflow problem of nanofluid that occurs during nanofluid infusion in breast tissue is simulated. The sensitivity of amplitude and frequency of the AMF is investigated on the tumor heating. The mesh-dependent solution of PBHTM is investigated. The simulated results show the success of breast cancer therapy incorporating MNPs with minimum normal cell damage. The validation of our simulation results with that of preexisting experimental studies is evident for our successful therapy. The increase in the frequency and amplitude of the AMF increased the temperature of the tumor. The change of mesh from coarser to finer increased the temperature through very small fractions. The magnetic flux density generated by the current-carrying coil conductors around the breast cup, the magnetic vector potential, and the temperature distribution inside the breast cup due to heating have been simulated.

Fifth, the enhanced permeation and retention (EPR) effect of nanofluid flowing from a blood vessel to the tumor through epithelial cell spacing, then its diffusion in the tumor interstitium, have been simulated using COMSOL Multiphysics. A 2D geometry of a porous tumor along with a blood vessel and epithelial cells is constructed. Nanofluid flows in the blood vessel and its diffusion in the tumors have been simulated and analyzed using FEM-based models of Navier-Stokes equations and the convection-diffusion equation. The simulation results show that the velocity of the nanofluid along the cross-section of the blood vessel follows the parabolic shape. Moreover, the velocity is higher in the blood vessel, and it decreases slowly while moving through epithelial spacing to the tumor interstitium. The mesh-dependent velocity analysis implies that the extremely fine mesh mode generates a better solution. The concentration of the nanofluid is higher near the blood vessel and decreases in moving away from the blood vessel to the tumor interstitium.

Sixth, the behavior of the diffusion of nanofluid flow around Happel's sphere has been simulated. The FEM-based models for the Navier-Stokes equation and the convection-diffusion equation are used to simulate the velocity and concentration for the nanofluid of biocompatible Fe_3O_4 MNPs around this structural unit in the porous tumor matrix. The mesh-dependent velocity of the nanofluid is analyzed quantitatively. The finer the mesh, the better the solution with a minor addition to the velocity. The velocity and concentration of nanofluid through the porous cubic and hexagonal structures of the porous tumor are also simulated. The simulation results show that the velocity of nanofluid through voids is a maximum and the flow-through of the cubical structure is smoother than the hexagonal structure. The flow is more turbulent and faster in the porous hexagonal structure. Next, the reacting nanofluid of blood and nanofluid has also been simulated while flowing through porous tumor. The corresponding concentrations before and after reaction has been analyzed quantitatively.

Lastly, the optimization in MFH has also been dealt with through standard optimization tools. The hyperthermia of cylindrical tumors through steady-state and transient analysis has been analyzed. The simulated steady-state temperature is validated with the analytical model in good agreement. The transient temperature curve is optimized with experimental data for the best fit and thermal conductivity is estimated for this fitting.

This research will aid in hyperthermia treatment planning in clinical applications. It will assist researchers in treatment protocols in clinical liver, brain, and breast cancer therapies and

Introduction

preexperimental in vivo and in vitro studies. It will aid therapeutic protocols and real-time clinical breast cancer therapies. It will also help in planning the infusion and diffusion of nanofluid before heat generation in hyperthermia treatment of cancer patients. Moreover, in the third world countries, where this treatment modality is in its infancy, this research will greatly assist clinicians in the effective planning of pre- and post hyperthermia treatment outcomes.

CHAPTER 1

Basics of magnetic fluid hyperthermia

1.1 What is nanoscience and nanotechnology?

Nanoscience is the understanding of nature at the microscale and nanotechnology is its application to instigate new devices, tools, and products. Nanotechnology is now an active research area that has made tremendous progress in both the industrial and economic zones in the present century. It has brought a revolution in the field of natural science, engineering sector, telecommunication, electronics, construction, textile industry, telecommunications, and medicine. Its particular applications in medicine include drug delivery to targeted sites in the body, transplantations of biocompatible nanomaterial, bone and tissue engineering, lab-on-chip biosensors for cancer diagnosis, and treatments [1–3]. Nanotechnology is incorporated in biomedical applications that aim at revolutionizing recent diagnosing and therapeutic modalities [4]. It is a multidisciplinary research field. It has created monosensors and nanoprobes of submicron-sized dimensions that are suitable for biological measurements. MNPs with diverse applications always remain interesting. At the nanoscale, their large surface area-to-volume ratio causes them to demonstrate the unique properties that make them more desirable [5,6]. The core theme of nanoscience and nanotechnology started after December 29, 1959 in a historical talk entitled "There's plenty of room in the bottom" by Richard Feynman during a meeting held at the California Institute of Technology Later, the term "Nanotechnology" was coined by Nario Taniguchi in 1974 during a scientific conference.

1.2 Basic types of biological experiments

All the experiments can be classified into three main types: in vitro, in vivo, and in silico experiments [7–10]. Each category possesses some advantages and limitations. These types are briefly explained below.

1.2.1 The in vitro studies

In vitro is a Latin word that means "within the glass." It is a method of conducting experiments within controlled surroundings and outside of the living species. The main limitations of such experiments include: (1) they do not succeed in replicating the precise cellular conditions of an organism, (2) about 99.6% of human microbiota species cannot be determined using in vitro studies, and (3) molecular concentration, especially their use in nuclear receptors. The study of bacteria, animals, and human cells in culture is referred to as in vitro study.

1.2.2 The in vivo studies

In vivo is a Latin word that means "within the living." In this type of experimentation, experiments are performed using the whole living organisms rather than partial or dead organisms. Clinical studies and animal studies come into this category. In vivo studies are better than in vitro studies to search for the overall performance of experiments on living subjects. These studies present an inclusive analysis of the nature of medicines and diseases. The clinical trials conducted to investigate the efficacy of an experimental drug comes into this category.

1.2.3 The in silico studies

In silico is a Latin word that means "Performed on the computer or via computer simulations." This term was publicly used for the first time in 1989 in a seminar held in Los Alamos in New Mexico, titled "Cellular Automata: Theory and Applications" by Pedro Miramontes. He is a well-known mathematician and is associated with the "National Autonomous University of Mexico." He used the term in silico in his talk titled "DNA and RNA Physiochemical constraints, Cellular Automata and Molecular Evolution" to demonstrate biological experimentation performed on the computer. This study opened a new horizon in research, and it mostly deals with how drugs interact with the body.

1.3 Fundamental types of cancer and its statistics

Cancer is the uncontrolled growth of abnormal cells in the body. It is a fatal disease and is a prominent cause of death globally, especially in low-income countries. According to *Cancer Research UK*, depending on the type of cells, cancer has the following main types: Carcinomas (skin cancer), Sarcomas (bone cancer), Leukemias (cancer of red blood cells), Lymphomas, Myelomas (cancer of the immune system), brain and spinal cord cancers. The International Agency for Research on Cancer (IARC) estimated 12.7 million new cancer cases and 7.6 million deaths globally in 2008. Hence, by the end of 2030, there would be 21.4 million new cancer cases and about 13.2 million deaths [11]. In 2012, WHO estimated 14 million cancer cases and about 8.2 million deaths [12].

1.4 Traditional techniques used for cancer treatment

Radiotherapy, chemotherapy, surgery, and immunotherapy are the currently used traditional treatment methods. Each of these therapeutic tool possesses some drawbacks.

1.4.1 Chemotherapy

Chemotherapy utilizes drugs to kill the tumor, but it also damages the surrounding normal tissue of the body. It uses powerful chemicals to kill the fast growth of cancer cells. It uses anticancer drugs as a part of standardized chemotherapy regimen. The treatment through chemotherapy might cause hair loss, anemia, infection, and loss of appetite. It has potential to completely remove the cancer. Lung cancer, Leukemia, ovarian cancers are generally required chemotherapy.

1.4.2 Radiotherapy

In Radiotherapy, the surrounding normal tissue of the body is also damaged due to the imperfection of targeting the tumor region only using radiations. It uses ionizing radiation radiations to kill tumor cells. At low doses it is used as X-Ray to see inside your body The patient feels buzzing during the treatment and he may feel some smell from machine. Radiation beam changes DNA makeup of tumor and causes it to shrink.

1.4.3 Surgery

Surgery is impractical for tumors that are located in the body at depth. This type of treatment is applied to the mass tumor that has gained some geometrical shape. It also termed as "Resection." The treatment time is very lengthy and can span over 8–12 h. Being the main type of treatment modality, the tumor can be completely treated, if the whole tumor is removed.

1.4.4 Immunotherapy

In immunotherapy, the body's natural system is boosted to fight against tumor cells. Natural killer cells and CD8+ cells play an important role in this regard. If the immune system is weak, the tumor cells grow without any hindrance. This treatment modality can produce effective results in some patients but may not be effective in some patients. The response rate ranges from 15% to 20%. It provides long-term protection against tumors. Using this treatment lung patients can live at least 5 years more.

Due to above stated drawbacks, clinicians researched other treatment techniques, where MFH has proved to be the best one [13]. This novel technique raised the temperature above 43°C of the tumor with minimum side effects. It has the potential to overcome these drawbacks [14]. It proved efficient for bladder cancer, cervical cancer, recurrent breast cancer, malignant melanoma, sarcoma of soft tissue, and deep-seated tumors [15–19]. The schematic representation of major types of cancer treatment modalities is demonstrated in Fig. 1.1 [20].

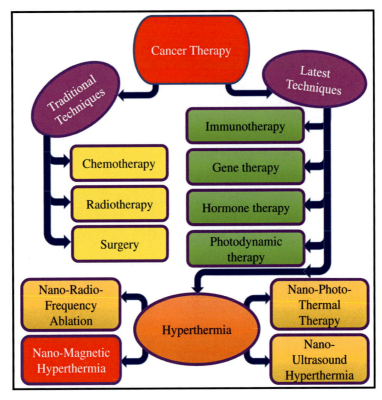

Fig. 1.1
Classification of cancer therapy into traditional and latest treatment techniques.

1.5 Hyperthermia

Historically, Egyptians used hyperthermia as a treatment tool about 5000years ago [21]. Now, it has gained more fame for cancer therapy. Internationally, it gained recognition in 1975 in an international congress held in Washington on hyperthermia oncology and later it became more famous [22]. The credit for the initiation of hyperthermia goes to Edwin Smith who used it for breast cancer therapy as mentioned in his surgical papyrus [23]. It is a therapeutic tool where the temperature of the tumor is raised to 45°C from 37°C of the body [24]. The basic methodology of this treatment modality is shown in Fig. 1.2.

1.6 Major types of hyperthermia

Thermotherapy can be classified into two major types: hyperthermia and thermal ablation. Depending on the temperature range of heating, hyperthermia can be classified into the following major categories.

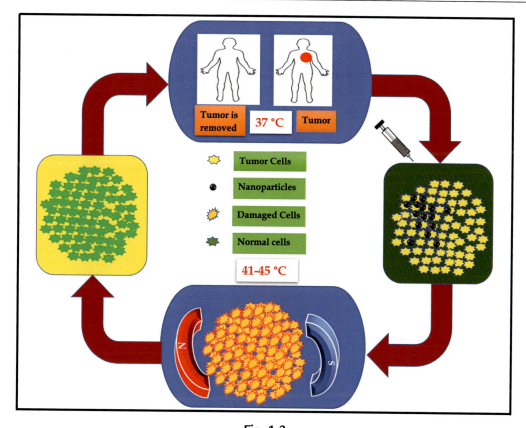

Fig. 1.2
A schematic cycle representation for the planning of MNP-induced hyperthermia for cancer therapy.

1.6.1 Moderate or mild hyperthermia

Moderate hyperthermia ranges from 41°C to 46°C and causes tumor damage under denaturation of the protein. It may also range from 42°C to 45°C [25].

1.6.2 Ablation hyperthermia

Thermal ablation ranges from 46°C to 56°C in which tumor cells are damaged following coagulation or carbonization or direct tissue damage [26].

1.6.3 Diathermia

Diathermia heats the tumor with a temperature $T < 41°C$.

Depending on the tumor location, hyperthermia is further divided into the following types.

1.6.4 Local hyperthermia

The main goal of using this treatment technique is to kill tumor cells while keeping healthy cells unharmed. Local hyperthermia stresses on selective heating of the tumor. That's why this technique attracted the worldwide community [13,27].

1.6.5 Regional hyperthermia

Regional hyperthermia deals with the heating of organs and body tissue.

1.6.6 Whole-body hyperthermia

Whole-body hyperthermia treats metastatic cancer cells. Whole-body hyperthermia was used as a heated blanket and immersion water baths in the 1960s. But it can generate many side effects and therefore it has to be neglected and the remaining two types should took the place [28].

1.6.7 Interstitial hyperthermia

Interstitial hyperthermia uses microwave antennas, rods, and needle electrodes to heat the tumor where heat is generated by microwaves. This tool showed success in the therapy of kidney, liver, bone, breast, and lung tissue [29].

1.7 Magnetic nanoparticles (MNPs) and hyperthermia

MNPs are well-known nanomaterials used in medicine. At the nanoscale (1–100 nm), nanomaterials demonstrate unique chemical, biological, and physical properties. The implementation and control of magnetic properties is the practical application of MNPs in cancer diagnosis and treatment. Its theory involves the synthesis of unconventional and core-shell MNPs. MNPs have shown diverse applications in the separation process, magnetic resonance imaging, and hyperthermia depending on their composition, size, structure, and physicochemical properties [30–32]. Mostly iron oxide, Mn, Co, Ni, Mg, Fe, Zn, and Gd MNPs and their oxides are used in hyperthermia. For example, Fe_3O_4 MNPs stabilized by dextran, cationic liposomes, hydrogel, and polyvinyl alcohol, and maghemite γ-Fe_2O_3 stabilized by ligand dextran are generally used in hyperthermia [33–36]. Among ferrites are cobalt ferrites ($CoFe_2O_3$), nickel ferrites ($NiFe_2O_4$), manganese ferrites ($MnFe_2O_4$), and lithium ferrites ($Li_{0.5}Fe_{2.5}O_4$) [37]. Both maghemite (γ-Fe_2O_3) and magnetite (Fe_3O_4) being nontoxic and biocompatible are used for heat generation [38], but with respect to cytotoxicity, these are inferior to the titanium, gold, and silver MNPs [39]. Maghemite is synthesized using an oxidation process at 300°C and magnetite MNPs are generated with typical sizes of 5 to 15 nm. Superparamagnetic magnetite MNPs were considered to be the best MNPs for MFH with a typical size of 11–13 nm [30]. By considering the parameters and MNP's chain size, the MNP's

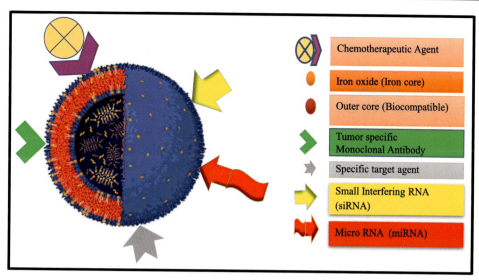

Fig. 1.3
Schematic diagram of iron oxide MNP with possible legends on the right side.

optimum size for hyperthermia was found to be 30% smaller than the one discovered previously [40]. Neutral granulocytes or macrophages can eat iron oxide MNPs in a natural way and these are ultimately degraded in lysosomes. These are turned into normal iron metabolism in the degradation process and eliminated from the body [41]. Iron oxide is capable of generating MFH, and therefore it is considered to be the best biomaterial for hyperthermia [42]. A schematic diagram of iron oxide MNP is presented in Fig. 1.3.

The iron-cobalt and ferrite core-shell MNPs possess better heating properties. The iron-cobalt MNPs have a higher specific power loss (SLP) due to higher saturation magnetization [43]. It was observed that the maghemite, magnetite, and iron-platinum MNPs were better than barium-ferrite, cobalt-ferrite, and iron-cobalt MNPs due to heating efficiency [44]. Generally, MNPs of size 10–50 nm are applied in biomedical applications. They demonstrate superparamagnetic behavior in this range with a large magnetic moment above block temperature. The MNPs used in hyperthermia should be stable with large heating power. Generally, these MNPs have five properties: (a) magnetic interactions, (b) geometrical properties, (c) interactions between the MNPs and the matrix material, (d) interparticle interactions, and (e) particle AMF interactions [45].

1.8 Synthesis of MNPs

Recently, enough research has been conducted to synthesize the MNPs focusing on stability, monodispersed, and shape control. These are synthesized with the expectation of property control, reproducibility, and uniformity [46]. Various synthesis techniques for the development of quality MNPs are demonstrated in Fig. 1.4 [47]. We will throw light on the synthesis of those MNPs which we are going to use in our simulations.

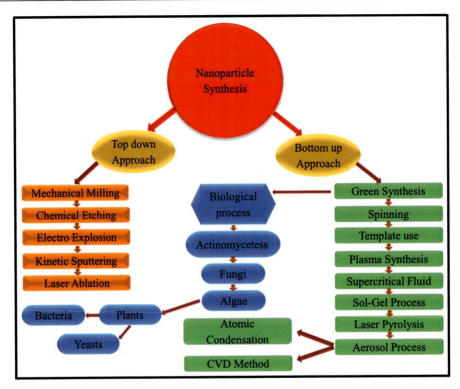

Fig. 1.4
Basic synthesis techniques of MNPs.

1.8.1 Synthesis of CoFe$_2$O$_4$@MnFe$_2$O$_4$ MNPs through modification of growth method

The core-shell CoFe$_2$O$_4$@MnFe$_2$O$_4$ MNPs are constituted by a 3-nm coating of MnFe$_2$O$_4$ and a 9-nm core of CoFe$_2$O$_4$ MNPs, yielding a 15-nm core-shell MNP, CoFe$_2$O$_4$@MnFe$_2$O$_4$. The synthesis was made according to reference [48] through the modification of the growth method. In this method, a 9-nm CoFe$_2$O$_4$ nanoparticle serves as the seed and MnFe$_2$O$_4$ is overgrown on the surface of the seed using the method of thermal decomposition. Fe(acac)$_3$ (5 mmol) and MnCl$_2$ (3.25 mmol) are put in a 250-mL round three-neck bottom flask in the presence of oleylamine, oleic acid, and trioctylamine. After that 9-nm CoFe$_2$O$_4$ MNPs suspended in hexane are injected and the mixture reaction is heated for 1h at 365°C. The heat source is removed and reaction products are cooled down to room temperature. The 15-nm size CoFe$_2$O$_4$@MnFe$_2$O$_4$ core-shell MNPs are isolated to use. A typical core-shell MNP is represented in Fig. 1.5.

1.8.2 Synthesis of Fe$_3$O$_4$ MNPs by the method of Molday

Fe$_3$O$_4$ MNPs were synthesized using the method of Molday [49]. The reactant's concentrations and precipitation temperature were varied to produce MNPs by coprecipitation. It was dried at 50°C to convert into powder under vacuum. Later it was dissolved with deionized water and

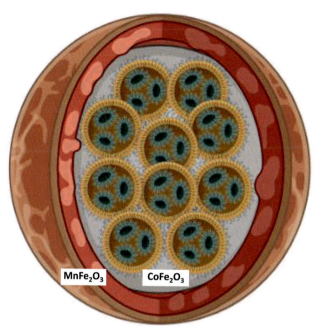

Fig. 1.5
A typical core-shell MNP.

sodium oleic acid. The aggregation was heated at 80°C for approximately 2h. These MNPs with a covering layer of oleic acid were dispersed in octane, benzene, toluene, and styrene in an ultrasonic generator to get a series of nanofluids. JEM-100, JEOL CO., Ltd., Japan was utilized to determine the size and shape of these MNPs. The size of the MNPs was determined using a Zetasizer (HPP5001).

1.8.3 Synthesis of Fe_3O_4 MNPs by facile method

Following this method, 1 mmol of citric acid, trisodium salt dihydrate ($C_6H_5Na_3O_7 \cdot 2H_2O$), $NaNO_3$ (0.2 mol), and 4 mmol of NaOH are mixed in 19 mL deionized water. The mixture is heated to 100°C and the pellucid solution is obtained. A further addition to this mixture was 1-mL of 2-M $FeSO_4 \cdot 4H_2O$ (2 mmol). The mixture was heated for 1 h at 100°C. The whole mixture was cooled down to room temperature. The Fe_3O_4 MNPs were obtained using a magnet after separation from the solvent. Black precipitation was redissolved in water for several minutes using an ultrasonic water bath. Using experimental parameters, the size of MNPs can be varied from ~20 to ~40 nm. The obtained MNPs with size 20 nm were stable for 1 month in water. The MNPs may be dispersed again in water after getting dried in the form of powder for a few weeks [50].

1.9 Loading MNPs at the tumor site

The MNPs can be loaded at the tumor sites in two ways, either intravenously or through a direct needle approach. We will briefly explain both approaches.

1.9.1 Intravenous injection approach

MNPs of size <10 nm can infiltrate through endothelial cell spacing to reach the tumor interstitium because these have gaps of 4μm as shown in Fig. 1.6. The lymphatic drainage of the tumor compels the MNPs to be collected at the tumor site. This phenomenon is known as "enhanced permeability and retention effect" (EPR) that distinguishes normal tissues from the cytotoxicity of the tumor. It is the collection of leaky blood vessels of the tumor. This is due to angiogenic regulators with enlarged gap junctions among endothelial cells and variations in lymphatic drainage. MNPs moved to the tumor location and converted into vesicles, endosomes, and lysosomes because of the existence of targeting legends. MNPs of sizes <25 nm can penetrate through the endothelium, but particles with size >50 nm collected in the liver [51]. Such MNPs took a long time to reach the tumor interstitium [52].

1.9.2 Direct needle injection approach

In this approach, MNPs are injected using Gauge needles, and generally an amount of 20–80 mg/cm^3 causes ablation up to 50°C [53]. But the needle approach causes tumor incongruence and invasiveness. It usually leaves untreated regions where the tumor can regrow. In contrast, the EPR effect efficiently loads tumors, but this technique gives unrequired concentration in the tumors

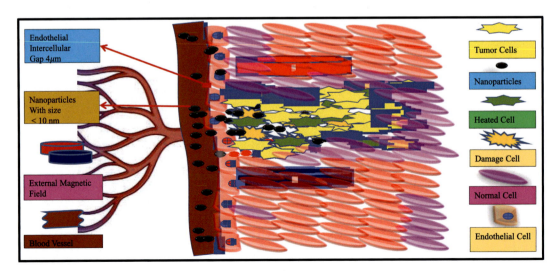

Fig. 1.6
Infiltration of MNPs to the tumor interstitium through endothelial cells and destruction mechanism.

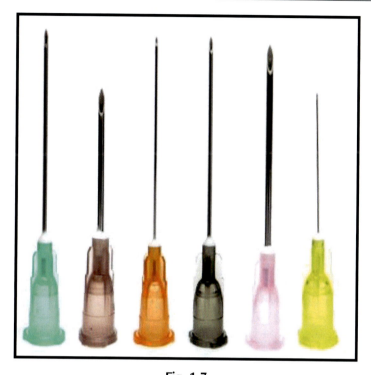

Fig. 1.7
Six hypodermic needles from bottom to top: 19-G×1.5″ (1.1×40mm), 20-G×1.5″ (0.9×40mm), 21-G×1.5″ (0.8×40mm), 22-G×1.25″ (0.7×30mm), 25-G×0.625″ (0.5×16mm), and 26-G×0.5″ (0.45×12mm).

before the process of systemic toxicity [54]. In the needle approach, the needles of different Gauges with different dimensions can be used to inject the MNPs in the tumor depending on the nature of the tumor. Generally, a needle of size 15-gauge with an inner radius of 1.372mm, an outer radius of 1.829mm, and having a wall thickness of 0.229mm is used to inject the nanofluid in the tumor. The dimension of different gauge needles can be found in Ref. [55]. The six needles with varying dimensions commonly used for medical purposes are demonstrated in Fig. 1.7.

1.10 Types of flow

There are different types of fluid flow as shown below [56] that will be used in the upcoming chapters.

1.10.1 Steady and unsteady flow

The general characteristics of the fluids are velocity, density, and pressure. If these characteristics do not change with time, the fluid flow is a steady flow. There are fluids where these characteristics change with time; such fluids are called unsteady fluids.

1.10.2 Uniform and nonuniform flow

When the fluid velocity is along the length of the direction of flow, the flow is termed as uniform. Here the velocity of the flow does not change from space to space at any given time. But in a nonuniform flow, the velocity of the flow changes from space to space at any given time.

1.10.3 Laminar and turbulent flow

When the particles of flow move along the straight streamlines, the flow is called laminar flow. The Reynolds number for such flows is generally less than 2000. On the other hand, when the fluid particles move in zigzag paths, it results in a turbulent flow that forms eddies. The Reynolds number for such flow is greater than 4000. For the Reynolds number between 2000 and 4000, the state of the fluid is called the transition state.

1.10.4 Compressible and incompressible flow

In compressible flows, the density changes from point to point in the fluid, whereas the density remains constant in incompressible flows.

1.10.5 Rotational and irrotational flows

There are some fluids where the fluid particles rotate about their own axis while moving along the streamline; these fluids are known as rotational flow. When the fluid particles do not rotate about their own axis, the fluid flow is termed irrotational flow.

1.10.6 One-, two-, and three-dimensional flow

When the fluid velocity is expressed as the function of one coordinate only and the other two coordinates are considered negligible, such flow is considered one-dimensional. The flow is two-dimensional if the velocity is a function of two coordinates and the third coordinate is negligible. In three-dimensional flows, the velocity is a function of three coordinates.

1.11 Blood vessels

The blood vessels are also termed channels that are responsible for carrying blood throughout your body. These beginning from the heart and ending again at the heart form a closed circuit. These are approximately 60,000 miles in length covering your whole body. These can be categorized into three main types, i.e., arteries, veins, and capillaries.

1.11.1 Arteries

These are responsible for carrying blood away from your heart. These are very strong muscular vessels and carry oxygenated blood to the body. These contribute 10%–15% of the body's blood. Arteries are further divided into arterioles. Both arteries and arterioles are flexible in structure. Their main function is to maintain blood pressure.

1.11.2 Veins

These are responsible for carrying blood back to your heart. They carry large volumes of deoxygenated blood back to your heart. Being fewer in number, these elastic veins can handle low blood pressure. Some veins have valves that open and close during the handling of blood flow. About 75% of blood is in your veins.

1.11.3 Capillaries

These are much smaller in diameter and connect arteries and veins. Being tiny, blood vessels act as thin walls between blood and tissue and organs. The wastage is pulled out through capillaries. The exchange of oxygen and carbon dioxide occurs in capillaries [57].

References

[1] Bañobre-López M, Pineiro-Redondo Y, De Santis R, Gloria A, Ambrosio L, Tampieri A, et al. Poly (caprolactone) based magnetic scaffolds for bone tissue engineering. J Appl Phys 2011;109:07B313.
[2] Tampieri A, D'Alessandro T, Sandri M, Sprio S, Landi E, Bertinetti L, et al. Intrinsic magnetism and hyperthermia in bioactive Fe-doped hydroxyapatite. Acta Biomater 2012;8:843–51.
[3] Gloria A, Russo T, d'Amora U, Zeppetelli S, d'Alessandro T, Sandri M, et al. Magnetic poly (ε-caprolactone)/iron-doped hydroxyapatite nanocomposite substrates for advanced bone tissue engineering. J R Soc Interface 2013;10:20120833.
[4] Hartung G, Mansoori G. In vivo General Trends, Filtration and Toxicity of Nanoparticles. J Nanomater Mol Nanotechnol 2: 3 2013;21:17–22.
[5] Guo S, Li D, Zhang L, Li J, Wang E. Monodisperse mesoporous superparamagnetic single-crystal magnetite nanoparticles for drug delivery. Biomaterials 2009;30:1881–9.
[6] Willard M, Kurihara L, Carpenter E, Calvin S, Harris V. Chemically prepared magnetic nanoparticles. Int Mater Rev 2004;49:125–70.
[7] Tunev SS, Hastey CJ, Hodzic E, Feng S, Barthold SW, Baumgarth N. Lymphoadenopathy during Lyme borreliosis is caused by spirochete migration-induced specific B cell activation. PLoS Pathog 2011;7, e1002066.
[8] Relman DA. Detection and identification of previously unrecognized microbial pathogens. Emerg Infect Dis 1998;4:382.
[9] Kinnings SL, Liu N, Buchmeier N, Tonge PJ, Xie L, Bourne PE. Drug discovery using chemical systems biology: repositioning the safe medicine Comtan to treat multi-drug and extensively drug resistant tuberculosis. PLoS Comput Biol 2009;5, e1000423.
[10] Roberts E, Magis A, Ortiz JO, Baumeister W, Luthey-Schulten Z. Noise contributions in an inducible genetic switch: a whole-cell simulation study. PLoS Comput Biol 2011;7, e1002010.
[11] American Cancer Society. Global cancer facts & figures. Atlanta: American Cancer Society; 2011.

[12] International Agency for Research on Cancer. IARC: Outdoor air pollution a leading environmental cause of cancer deaths. International Agency for Research on Cancer; 2011.
[13] Habash RW, Bansal R, Krewski D, Alhafid HT. Thermal therapy, part 2: hyperthermia techniques. Crit Rev Biomed Eng 2006;34:491–542.
[14] Kobayashi T. Cancer hyperthermia using magnetic nanoparticles. Biotechnol J 2011;6:1342–7.
[15] van der Zee J, González D, van Rhoon GC, van Dijk JD, van Putten WL, Hart AA. Comparison of radiotherapy alone with radiotherapy plus hyperthermia in locally advanced pelvic tumours: a prospective, randomised, multicentre trial. Lancet 2000;355:1119–25.
[16] Overgaard J, Bentzen S, Gonzalez DG, Hulshof M, Arcangeli G, Dahl O, et al. Randomised trial of hyperthermia as adjuvant to radiotherapy for recurrent or metastatic malignant melanoma. Lancet 1995;345:540–3.
[17] International Collaborative Hyperthermia Group, Vernon CC, Hand JW, Field SB, Machin D, Whaley JB, et al. Radiotherapy with or without hyperthermia in the treatment of superficial localized breast cancer: results from five randomized controlled trials. Int J Radiat Oncol Biol Phys 1996;35:731–44.
[18] Issels RD, Lindner LH, Verweij J, Wust P, Reichardt P, Schem B-C, et al. Neo-adjuvant chemotherapy alone or with regional hyperthermia for localised high-risk soft-tissue sarcoma: a randomised phase 3 multicentre study. Lancet Oncol 2010;11:561–70.
[19] Colombo R, Salonia A, Leib Z, Pavone-Macaluso M, Engelstein D. Long-term outcomes of a randomized controlled trial comparing thermochemotherapy with mitomycin-C alone as adjuvant treatment for non-muscle-invasive bladder cancer (NMIBC). BJU Int 2011;107:912–8.
[20] Hehr T, Wust P, Bamberg M, Budach W. Current and potential role of thermoradiotherapy for solid tumours. Oncol Res Treat 2003;26:295–302.
[21] EJ H. Physical and biologic basis of radiation therapy. In: Moss' radiation oncology: Rationale, technique, results; 1994. p. 3–66.
[22] Dewey W, Hopwood L, Sapareto S, Gerweck L. Cellular responses to combinations of hyperthermia and radiation. Radiology 1977;123:463–74.
[23] Overgaard J, Gonzalez DG, Hulshof M, Arcangeli G, Dahl O, Mella O, et al. Hyperthermia as an adjuvant to radiation therapy of recurrent or metastatic malignant melanoma. A multicentre randomized trial by the European Society for Hyperthermic Oncology. Int J Hyperth 1996;12:3–20.
[24] Christophi C, Winkworth A, Muralihdaran V, Evans P. The treatment of malignancy by hyperthermia. Surg Oncol 1998;7:83–90.
[25] Fagnoni FF, Zerbini A, Pelosi G, Missale G. Combination of radiofrequency ablation and immunotherapy. Front Biosci 2008;13:369–81.
[26] Goldstein L, Dewhirst M, Repacholi M, Kheifets L. Summary, conclusions and recommendations: adverse temperature levels in the human body. Int J Hyperth 2003;19:373–84.
[27] Robins HI, Woods JP, Schmitt CL, Cohen JD. A new technological approach to radiant heat whole body hyperthermia. Cancer Lett 1994;79:137–45.
[28] Nielsen OS, Horsman M, Overgaard J. A future for hyperthermia in cancer treatment? Eur J Cancer 2001;37:1587–9.
[29] Lin JC, Wang Y-J. Interstitial microwave antennas for thermal therapy. Int J Hyperth 1987;3:37–47.
[30] Pankhurst QA, Connolly J, Jones S, Dobson J. Applications of magnetic nanoparticles in biomedicine. J Phys D Appl Phys 2003;36:R167.
[31] Laurent S, Forge D, Port M, Roch A, Robic C, Vander Elst L, et al. Magnetic iron oxide nanoparticles: synthesis, stabilization, vectorization, physicochemical characterizations, and biological applications. Chem Rev 2008;108:2064–110.
[32] Hadjipanayis CG, Bonder MJ, Balakrishnan S, Wang X, Mao H, Hadjipanayis GC. Metallic iron nanoparticles for MRI contrast enhancement and local hyperthermia. Small 2008;4:1925–9.
[33] Dennis C, Jackson A, Borchers J, Ivkov R, Foreman A, Hoopes P, et al. The influence of magnetic and physiological behaviour on the effectiveness of iron oxide nanoparticles for hyperthermia. J Phys D Appl Phys 2008;41, 134020.

[34] Kawai N, Futakuchi M, Yoshida T, Ito A, Sato S, Naiki T, et al. Effect of heat therapy using magnetic nanoparticles conjugated with cationic liposomes on prostate tumor in bone. Prostate 2008;68:784–92.

[35] Suto M, Hirota Y, Mamiya H, Fujita A, Kasuya R, Tohji K, et al. Heat dissipation mechanism of magnetite nanoparticles in magnetic fluid hyperthermia. J Magn Magn Mater 2009;321:1493–6.

[36] Lévy M, Wilhelm C, Siaugue J-M, Horner O, Bacri J-C, Gazeau F. Magnetically induced hyperthermia: size-dependent heating power of γ-Fe2O3 nanoparticles. J Phys Condens Matter 2008;20, 204133.

[37] Kim D-H, Lee S-H, Kim K-N, Kim K-M, Shim I-B, Lee Y-K. Temperature change of various ferrite particles with alternating magnetic field for hyperthermic application. J Magn Magn Mater 2005;293:320–7.

[38] Hergt R, Andra W, d'Ambly CG, Hilger I, Kaiser WA, Richter U, et al. Physical limits of hyperthermia using magnetite fine particles. IEEE Trans Magn 1998;34:3745–54.

[39] Koch CM, Winfrey AL. FEM optimization of energy density in tumor hyperthermia using time-dependent magnetic nanoparticle power dissipation. IEEE Trans Magn 2014;50:1–7.

[40] Branquinho LC, Carrião MS, Costa AS, Zufelato N, Sousa MH, Miotto R, et al. Effect of magnetic dipolar interactions on nanoparticle heating efficiency: implications for cancer hyperthermia. Sci Rep 2013;3:2887.

[41] Berry CC, Curtis AS. Functionalisation of magnetic nanoparticles for applications in biomedicine. J Phys D Appl Phys 2003;36:R198.

[42] Wang X, Gu H, Yang Z. The heating effect of magnetic fluids in an alternating magnetic field. J Magn Magn Mater 2005;293:334–40.

[43] Habib A, Ondeck C, Chaudhary P, Bockstaller M, McHenry M. Evaluation of iron-cobalt/ferrite core-shell nanoparticles for cancer thermotherapy. J Appl Phys 2008;103:07A307.

[44] Kappiyoor R, Liangruksa M, Ganguly R, Puri IK. The effects of magnetic nanoparticle properties on magnetic fluid hyperthermia. J Appl Phys 2010;108, 094702.

[45] Obaidat I, Issa B, Haik Y. Magnetic properties of magnetic nanoparticles for efficient hyperthermia. Nanomaterials 2015;5:63–89.

[46] Ito A, Shinkai M, Honda H, Kobayashi T. Medical application of functionalized magnetic nanoparticles. J Biosci Bioeng 2005;100:1–11.

[47] Iravani S. Green synthesis of metal nanoparticles using plants. Green Chem 2011;13:2638–50.

[48] Lee J-H, Jang J-t, Choi J-s, Moon SH, Noh S-h, Kim J-w, et al. Exchange-coupled magnetic nanoparticles for efficient heat induction. Nat Nanotechnol 2011;6:418.

[49] Molday RS. Magnetic iron-dextran microspheres. Google Patents; 1984.

[50] Hui C, Shen C, Yang T, Bao L, Tian J, Ding H, et al. Large-scale Fe_3O_4 nanoparticles soluble in water synthesized by a facile method. J Phys Chem C 2008;112:11336–9.

[51] Bergs JW, Wacker MG, Hehlgans S, Piiper A, Multhoff G, Roedel C, et al. The role of recent nanotechnology in enhancing the efficacy of radiation therapy. Biochim Biophys Acta Rev Cancer 2015;1856:130–43.

[52] Maeda H, Nakamura H, Fang J. The EPR effect for macromolecular drug delivery to solid tumors: improvement of tumor uptake, lowering of systemic toxicity, and distinct tumor imaging in vivo. Adv Drug Deliv Rev 2013;65:71–9.

[53] Hilger I, Rapp A, Greulich K-O, Kaiser WA. Assessment of DNA damage in target tumor cells after thermoablation in mice. Radiology 2005;237:500–6.

[54] van Landeghem FK, Maier-Hauff K, Jordan A, Hoffmann K-T, Gneveckow U, Scholz R, et al. Post-mortem studies in glioblastoma patients treated with thermotherapy using magnetic nanoparticles. Biomaterials 2009;30:52–7.

[55] Sakuma Y, Kishimoto N, Momota Y. Appropriate color codes for medical materials and devices in terms of color vision deficiency management to ensure patient safety. J Osaka Dent Univ 2017;51:31–8.

[56] Kumar S. Flow through open channels. In: Fluid mechanics, vol. 2. Springer; 2023. p. 397–419.

[57] Townsley MI. Structure and composition of pulmonary arteries, capillaries and veins. Compr Physiol 2012;2:675.

CHAPTER 2

Historical background of magnetic fluid hyperthermia

2.1 Mathematical modeling approach toward MFH

We can apply heat to the biological tissue up to a certain maximum limit of temperature which is tolerated by the tissue because heat is dissipated due to blood flow. If there is no flow of blood, the temperature of tissue will increase linearly with the time of heating at some specific heating rate. But if blood flows, the temperature will increase nonlinearly due to the dissipation of heat. The rate of the temperature rise will continuously decrease until it reaches a steady state. Therefore, BHTM is developed to account for the heat loss term arising from blood flow to describe the heat transfer in biological tissue [1,2]. In hyperthermia, temperature plays a central role, so it is extremely important to calculate the temperature field accurately inside the biological tissue. For this purpose, about 65 years ago, Penne in 1948 developed PBHTM [3] for heat transfer in biological tissue. In his work, he calculated the skin affected topography of temperature in the upper extremity using the gradient approach and he also determined the effect of blood flow on the proximal forearm. Additionally, simultaneous rectal, brachial arterial blood, and deep forearm temperature were measured. Also, temperature-depth distributions of steady-state tissue and the analytical theory of heat applied to evaluate the effects of local heat production along with calculating circulation were determined. This PBHTM was based on the Fourier law which says that the *"thermal disturbance move at infinite speed and small disturbance is felt instantaneously in the body."* Penne developed this model to study transfer heat in a resting human forearm considering the heat diffusion between the blood and adjacent tissues and also heat generation due to the metabolism in tissue. The BHTM developed by him is given by

$$c\rho \frac{\partial \eta}{\partial t} = -K\left[\frac{\partial^2 \eta}{\partial r^2} + \frac{1}{r}\frac{\partial \eta}{\partial r} + \frac{1}{r^2}\frac{\partial \eta}{\partial \phi} + \frac{\partial^2 \eta}{\partial z^2}\right] + Q_m + Q_b \qquad (2.1)$$

where η is the tissue temperature (K), r is normal to the cylindrical isothermal surface (cm), ρ is the tissue density (kg m^{-3}), c is the tissue-specific heat (J kg^{-1} K^{-1}), K is the tissue-specific thermal conductivity (W m^{-1} K^{-1}), Q_b is the rate of heat transfer from blood to tissue (Jm^{-3} s^{-1}), Q_m is the rate of heat production of tissue (Jm^{-3} s^{-1}), and for complete equilibrium between tissue and capillary blood, $Q_b = U\mu(\eta_a - \eta_v)$ where $U = \rho\mu$ is the volume of blood flow in tissue (g cm^{-3} s^{-1}), μ is the specific heat of blood (J kg^{-1} K^{-1}), η_a is the arterial blood temperature (K), and η_v is venous blood temperature (K). Based on certain assumptions, Penne neglected the gradient along the long axis of the forearm $\frac{\partial^2 \eta}{\partial z^2}$ and the angular gradient $\frac{\partial \eta}{\partial \varphi}$ was also taken to be zero due to circular symmetry. Moreover, he considered $Q_b = 0$ to be uniform throughout the cylinder. He solved the remaining equation analytically in the form of Bessel's equation of zeroth order. His analytical curve of temperature in the parabolic form agreed with the experimental curve obtained from the temperature distribution in the forearm. Since the PBHTM was based on certain assumptions, this model was therefore unable to address convective directional phenomena and exchange of heat between closely packed countercurrent vessels of blood. Therefore, this basic model has to be modified to overcome these shortcomings. Wulff [4] extended PBHTM by incorporating an impact of flow direction and proposed the corrected form of BHTM as represented by

$$c\rho_p \frac{\partial \eta}{\partial t} = -K\nabla^2 \eta - \rho_p \mu_b U_h + Q_m \tag{2.2}$$

where he took the metabolic reaction term $Q_m = \rho_b c_b \Delta H_f \nabla \varepsilon$ and $\eta = \eta_b$. Later, PBHTM was extended by Chen and Holmes [5], Weinbaum et al. [6,7], Balidemaj et al. [8], Deuflhard et al. [9], Nguyen et al. [10], and in work [11–18].

MFH of cancer treatment was first initiated in 1957 when Gilchrist et al. [19] used maghemite (γ-Fe$_2$O$_3$) MNPs to selectively heat the lymphatic nodes of dogs [20], and later Gordon et al. [21] in 1979 used a magnetite solution of dextran with 6 nm core sizes. LeBrun et al. [22] developed and performed a computer algorithm to export micro-CT images and to produce the tumor geometry and specific absorption rate (SAR) distribution for simulations of heat transfer in MNP-induced hyperthermia. They developed a rectangular column as geometry for the mouse body. They used PBHTM to simulate steady-state temperature inside the tumor and mouse body as described by the following equations:

$$c\rho \frac{\partial \eta}{\partial t} = 0 = -k_{\text{tumor}} \nabla^2 \eta_{\text{tumor}} + \text{SAR} + Q_{m,\text{tumor}} + \omega_{\text{tumor}} (\rho c)_{\text{blood}} (\eta_a - \eta_{\text{tumor}}) \tag{2.3}$$

$$c\rho \frac{\partial \eta}{\partial t} = 0 = k_t \nabla^2 \eta_t + Q_{m,t} + \omega_t (\rho c)_{\text{blood}} (\eta_a - \eta_t) \tag{2.4}$$

where the volumetric heat generation rate induced by MNPs was applied to the tumor region only. In another study, LeBrun et al. [23] designed a heating protocol to completely remove the PC3 tumor by applying MNP-induced hyperthermia in one session only. This was based on the micro-CT image developed in the tumor and mouse models. They again considered PBHTM for transient temperature distribution in tissue. They employed this model to both the mouse body and the tumor given by the following equations:

$$c_t \rho_t \frac{\partial \eta_t}{\partial t} = K_t \nabla^2 \eta_t + \omega_t \rho_b c_b (\eta_b - \eta_t) + Q_{met,t} \tag{2.5}$$

$$c_c \rho_c \frac{\partial \eta_c}{\partial t} = K_c \nabla^2 \eta_c + \omega_c \rho_b c_b (\eta_b - \eta_c) + Q_{met,c} + Q_{\text{MNP}} \qquad (2.6)$$

where Q_{MNP} is volumetric heat generation induced by MNPs which was applied only to the tumor region because MNPs are confined to the tumors. More explanation of this factor can be found in Ref. [24]. They determined the time to complete the tumor damage to be 25 min with the infusion rate of 3 μL/min. However, heating time is longer in the high infusion rates. Collateral thermal damage to the neighboring tissue was only acceptable in the infusion rate of 3 μL/min. From this research, they identified the injection strategy and heating protocols. Sankar and Zhang [25] studied the integrated therapy of X-ray radiation therapy and gold nanoparticle-induced hyperthermia for the treatment of cutaneous squamous carcinoma (CSC). Their governing bio-heat equations for both therapies are represented by the following equations:

$$\frac{\partial \eta}{\partial t} = D_{AB} \left[\frac{1}{r} \frac{\partial}{\partial r} \left(r \frac{\partial \eta}{\partial r} \right) + \frac{\partial^2 \eta}{\partial z^2} \right] + R_{\text{INJ}}, R_{\text{INJ}} = \frac{\left(\frac{1\,\text{mL}}{\text{min}} \cdot \frac{1\,\text{min}}{60\,\text{s}} \cdot \frac{100\,\text{mgAuNP}}{\text{mL}} \right)}{V_{\text{INJ}}} \qquad (2.7)$$

$$c_t \rho_t \frac{\partial \eta}{\partial t} = K_t \left[\frac{1}{r} \frac{\partial}{\partial r} \left(r \frac{\partial \eta}{\partial r} \right) + \frac{\partial^2 \eta}{\partial z^2} \right] + \omega_b c_b (\eta_b - \eta) + Q_m + Q_{\text{IR}}, Q_{\text{IR}} = \frac{0.015\,\text{W}\,\text{mm}^{-2}}{35\,\text{mm}} e^{\left(-\frac{(z-z_0)}{35\,\text{mm}} \right)}$$

$$(2.8)$$

where all terms in both equations have their usual meanings. They simulated these models on COMSOL Multiphysics and also optimized their combined therapy. They determined the optimized time to be 60s of heating using 1.5W/cm^2 infrared lamps and 0.35Gy. Moreover, the Gold MNP-induced hypertherapy model was validated with experimental work of Ref. [26], and the X-ray radiation therapy model was validated with the work of Ref. [27]. Eagle et al. [24] modeled three phenomena they (a) modeled the MNP-induced hyperthermia by incorporating particle diffusion, particle injection, and particle heating; (b) quantified the tissue necrosis extent during the heating process; (c) optimized the heating duration to maximize the tumor damage while minimizing the damage of normal tissue. They considered the tumor as a sphere surrounded by a larger sphere which was taken as normal tissue. MNPs were directly injected into the tumor with a needle. Then the external magnetic field was applied to produce heat due to the presence of MNPs in the tumor through relaxation effects that kill the tumor cells. Again, they considered the PBHTM to incorporate the effect of MNPs. Their developed model is represented by the equation

$$c\rho \frac{\partial \eta}{\partial t} = K \left[\frac{1}{r} \frac{\partial}{\partial r} \left(r \frac{\partial \eta}{\partial r} \right) + \frac{\partial^2 \eta}{\partial z^2} \right] + \rho_b c_b V_b (\eta - \eta_b) + Q_{np}, \quad Q_{np} = \pi \mu_0 \chi_0 H_0^2 f \left[\frac{\omega \tau}{1 + (\omega \tau)^2} \right]$$

$$(2.9)$$

They also validated their developed model with the Javidi et al. [28] model in two ways; firstly, they validated it with a computational model which revealed that it followed expected trends, and secondly they validated the tumor properties with agarose gel. The agreements were excellent. Moreover, using their formulation, the optimized heating time was obtained to be 11.5 min [29]. Salloum et al. [29] formulated a general algorithm to optimize a multiscale injection strategy. Firstly, PBHTM was used to evaluate the thermally affected region for an irregular shape the tumor developed in a normal tissue region. An initial guess of the multiple injection site locations and the associated SAR distribution was calculated. Secondly, PBHTM was applied to calculate temperature fields in normal tissue and the tumor region. Using the Nelder Mead Simplex Method for optimization and their developed model is given by

$$\frac{k}{r^2}\frac{\partial}{\partial r}\left(r^2 \frac{\partial \eta}{\partial r}\right) + \rho_b c_b \omega_b (\eta - \eta_b) + \text{SAR}, \quad \text{SAR} = A e^{\left(-\frac{r^2}{r_0^2}\right)} \tag{2.10}$$

The above model was then solved analytically for temperature distribution, η. The tumor was considered to be contained in cube. Assuming the thermal properties to be constant, the 3D PBHTM was developed in the following equation:

$$K\left[\frac{\partial^2 \eta}{\partial x^2} + \frac{\partial^2 \eta}{\partial y^2} + \frac{\partial^2 \eta}{\partial z^2}\right] + \rho_b c_b \omega_b (\eta - \eta_b) + Q_m + \sum_{i=1}^{M} A_i \cdot e^{\left(-\frac{r_i^2}{r_{0,i}^2}\right)} = 0 \tag{2.11}$$

where the last term represents the heat source produced near the vicinity of MNPs injection locations, heating occurs mainly in the tumor region, M represents the number of injections, and r_i is the radial distance from the injection site i and is modeled as

$$r_i^2 = (x - x_i)^2 + (x - y_i)^2 + (x - z_i)^2, \quad i = 1,2,3,\ldots M \tag{2.12}$$

Similar work was carried out by Hall et al. [30] to treat the tumor of irregular shape using 2D and 3D models to optimize injection locations to optimize the temperature. Their developed models in 2D and 3D are represented by the following equation.

$$K\left[\frac{\partial^2 \eta}{\partial x^2} + \frac{\partial^2 \eta}{\partial y^2}\right] + \sum_{i=1}^{n} Q_i = \frac{\partial \eta}{\partial t} \tag{2.13}$$

$$K\left[\frac{\partial^2 \eta}{\partial x^2} + \frac{\partial^2 \eta}{\partial y^2} + \frac{\partial^2 \eta}{\partial z^2}\right] + \sum_{i=1}^{n} Q_i = \frac{\partial \eta}{\partial t} \tag{2.14}$$

After validation of their model through simulation with analytical results, they successfully achieved their objectives. The applicability of PBHTM to biological tissues is limited due to physical assumptions. For instance, they considered only thermal equilibrium at capillaries and did not consider heat transfer between the skin and larger blood vessels. They have taken an infinite heat propagation rate because it was based on Fourier's law of thermal conduction. Moreover, they also took a homogeneous and isotropic volume. Perigo et al. [31] thought that these assumptions are met in real tissues and heterogeneities make them demonstrate a non-Fourier behavior that produces a thermal response lag on applying a temperature change. It means there is a heat relaxation time of the tissue, which may reach the value of ~100 s for certain biological materials due to the difference between heat propagation processes and the occurrence of the temperature gradient. This factor was incorporated in the dual-phase-lag equation of the namesake model, or the following hyperbolic bio-heat equation

$$\rho c \left[\tau \frac{\partial^2 \eta}{\partial t^2} + \frac{\partial \eta}{\partial t} \right] + \nabla \cdot (-k \nabla \eta) + \rho_b c_b (\eta - \eta_b) + Q_m + Q_{ext} + \tau \left(\omega_b c_b \frac{\partial \eta}{\partial t} + \frac{\partial Q_{ext}}{\partial t} + \frac{\partial Q_m}{\partial t} \right) \tag{2.15}$$

When $\tau \to 0$, the above equation reduces to PBHTM [3]. But despite its limitations, the PBHTM of heat transfer has been justified by many experimental studies [31]. In previous studies, there were certain parameters that were not considered while designing thermotherapy, and these parameters were the main barrier for implantation of MFH. Liangruksa et al. [32] investigated these parameters for idealized MFH and suggested an optimal strategy to minimize harm to normal tissue. They analyzed the steady and transient responses to the tumor and healthy tissue to MFH which may prove fruitful for in vitro and in vivo experiments. They considered the tumor to be of spherical in shape surrounded by healthy tissue. The tumor and healthy tissues have a specific blood perfusion rate and basal temperature. The thermal mechanism was carried out by taking into account the PBHM [3] in spherical coordinates to develop the following model:

$$\rho_t c_t \frac{\partial \eta_t}{\partial t} = \frac{K_t}{r^2} \left[\frac{\partial}{\partial r} \left(r^2 \frac{\partial \eta_t}{\partial r} \right) \right] - \dot{m}_b c_b (\eta_t - \eta_b) + P \tag{2.16}$$

They transformed this model into a dimensionless form

$$\frac{\partial \eta^*}{\partial t^*} = \nabla^{*2} \eta^* - P_e \eta^* + \frac{F_0}{J} \tag{2.17}$$

where $Pe = m_b' c_b (R^2/k_t)$ is the Peclet number, which represents the heat transport ratio due to convection to that by conduction, $J = \rho_t c_t \eta_b / \pi \mu_0 \chi H^2$ is the ratio of the joule heating energy, and $F_0 = \tau(\omega R)^2 / 2\pi \alpha_t (1 + (\omega \tau))^2$ is the Fourier number. These were three key parameters that affect the temperature distributions in the tumor and healthy tissue. Maenosono and Saita [33] revealed that FePt (MNPs) have a high-performance nanoheater for MFH because these were of high saturation magnetization, high Curie temperature, and high chemical stability. They applied the model based on PBHM [3] to develop the following model

$$\rho c_p \frac{\partial \eta}{\partial t} = \nabla k (\nabla \eta) + \rho_b c_b \omega_b (\eta_a - \eta) + Q_m + P \tag{2.18}$$

where $P = 3.97 \times 10^5$ W/m^3 for FCC FePt MNPs and $P = 1.95 \times 10^5$ W/m^3 for magnetite MNPs. To calculate heat generation and heat transfer in the tissue when MNPs were administered in the tumor, they comparatively studied the performances of magnetite, maghemite, FeCo, and

L10-phase FePt MNPs and concluded that FCC FePt MNPs have the superior ability in MFH. In a study, Liu and Chen [34] raised the temperature in biological tissues in hypertherapy by utilizing a dual-phase lag model which revealed the local nonequilibrium on thermal behavior. The tumor was considered to be a solid sphere surrounded by normal tissue. The impact of the time lag, blood perfusion rate, rate of metabolic heat generation, and other parameters of tissue was investigated. They incorporated the following linearized dual-phase-lag model:

$$\tau_q \frac{\partial q}{\partial t} + q = -k\frac{\partial \eta}{\partial r} - k\tau_\eta \frac{\partial^2 \eta}{\partial t \partial r} \qquad (2.19)$$

into the PBHTM to develop their model:

$$\rho c \frac{\partial \eta}{\partial t} = -\frac{\partial q}{\partial r} - \frac{2}{r}q + \rho_b c_b \omega_b (\eta_a - \eta) + Q_m + Q_r \qquad (2.20)$$

Describing temperature distribution in the tumor and tissue regions subjected to some B.Cs. Wu et al. [35] also solved the model of MFH by considering the tumor in a spherical shape with promising results. Branquinho et al. [36] proposed a model obeying dipole interactions. The optimized particle sizes predicted for hyperthermia from that model were about 30% smaller than those previously developed, depending on the nanoparticle parameters and chain size. Moreover, optimum chain lengths depend on the surface-to-surface distance of MNPs. Rast and Harrison [37] developed a computational model for MFH by incorporating the solution of Maxwell's equation in the tumor model and tissue as a solution to the PBHTM. They solved both models using FDM and demonstrated that there exists an enhanced tissue temperature near the center of the tumor for a low tumor blood perfusion rate. Feng et al. [38] constructed an adaptive finite element tumor model:

$$\rho c \frac{\partial \eta}{\partial t} = \nabla \cdot (k \nabla \eta) + c_b \omega_b (\eta_a - \eta) + Q, \quad Q = 3P\mu_{atot}\mu_{tr} e^{\left(-\frac{\mu_{eff}(r-r_0)}{4\pi(r-r_0)}\right)} \qquad (2.21)$$

This model was able to predict the temperature distribution and damage due to laser therapy in prostate cancer with and without the inclusion of nanoshells. Nanoshell-induced laser therapy increased the energy deposition in the tumor, enhancing the tissue damage and reduction of power required for the tumor damage. Additionally, this model can be used to obtain optimal hyperthermia protocols concerning both temperature and cell death distribution. With mature nanoshell injections and a reliable computational model, the output of laser therapy for cancer treatment will become more predictable and controllable. Kurgan studied the energy absorption of MNPs in hyperthermia. He developed his model (2.22) based on the PBHTM described below under a steady-state condition and solved it to determine the temperature distributions inside the tumor and surrounding tissues

$$0 = \nabla \cdot (k \nabla \eta) + \rho_b c_b \omega_b (\eta_a - \eta) + Q_{eddy} + Q_{met} + W_s, \quad W_s = \frac{2f(\pi R B_m)^2 \sigma}{3} \qquad (2.22)$$

The heat release due to the blood circulation was also considered. Numerical results were presented for heat generated by ferromagnetic NPs in order to minimize the negative effects of radiofrequency radiation. Bellizzi et al. [39] in another study numerically assessed the criteria for optimizing the operative conditions in MFH on a human head realistic model. After applying this criterion for the brain, the tumors revealed that the acceptable values for the product between magnetic field amplitude and frequency may be 2–4 times larger than the safety threshold of $4.85 \times 10^8 \, \text{Am}^{-1} \, \text{s}^{-1}$. This would lead to a reduction of dosage of MNPs required for efficient therapy.

Pearce et al. [40] analyze numerically the MNPs induced the tumor heating experiment [41]. They utilized the PBHTM to develop their model (Eq. 2.23)

$$\rho_t c_t \frac{\partial \eta}{\partial t} = \nabla \cdot (k \nabla \eta) + \rho_b c_b \omega_b (\eta - \eta_a) + Q_{gen} + Q_{met}, \quad Q_{gen} = \omega \ddot{\mu} |H|^2 \qquad (2.23)$$

Tools for effective heating are the minimum loading of iron oxide required to achieve adequate heating, bio-distribution of magnetic materials, and targeted magnetic field strengths. These criteria determine the validation of this tool toward tumor treatment. Efficient heating of surface of the tumors (5–10 mm) requires an efficient tumor loading. There is a prominent treatment design parameter that establishes a useful treatment planning for the distribution of MNPs. Huang et al. [42], firstly used extended gold nanorods (GNRs) in hyperthermia for human prostate tumor and irradiated GNRs by laser. This model successfully demonstrated the temperature distribution for various laser irradiation and optical density levels. They also presented the cellular death model $k = Ae^{-Ea/RT}$ based on the Arrhenius injury model [43]. This model also predicted cell death levels that were in good agreement with experimental results. In another identical study to the above, Elliot et al. [44] analytically solved the laser-induced thermal therapy for the treatment of cancer and modeled the resulting temperature distribution for treatment planning. They demonstrated that the efficiency of laser-induced thermal therapy can be enhanced with the presence of gold-coated Nanoshells. The Nanoshells are forced to exhibit a surface plasmonic resonance at the frequency of operating laser light. It dramatically increased the efficiency of the laser treatment. Secondly, Huang et al. [45] determined the minimum temperature for photothermal destruction of the tumor cells integrated with Gold NPs. They developed a mathematical model for this combined therapy represented by

$$c\rho \frac{\partial \eta}{\partial t} = \frac{k}{r^2} \frac{\partial}{\partial r} \left(r^2 \frac{\partial \eta}{\partial r} \right) + Q_s, \quad Q_s = Q(1 - 10^{-A}) \qquad (2.24)$$

where A is the optical density or absorbance of gold NPs and Q (W/m^3) is the incident laser power. This treatment modality that used much lower laser power than needed for healthy cells was proved to be very effective. Xu et al. [46] used arterial embolization hyperthermia (AEH) to determine the heat distribution by simulation of the external ferrite core applicator and SAR of MNPs in the maghemite-gelled composite model. They proposed the following model:

$$\rho c \frac{\partial \eta}{\partial t} = \nabla \cdot (k \nabla \eta) + c_b \omega_b (\eta_a - \eta) + Q_r, \quad Q_r = \mathrm{SAR}(x, y, z) \cdot \xi_{Fe}(x, y, z) \qquad (2.25)$$

where they took Q_r of the bulk tissue unit to further formulate their model. The theoretical results were in good agreement with the experimental results. Nabil and Zunino [47] studied MFH collaborated with a novel model arising from mass, flow, and heat transport in biological tissues and is known as an *embedded multiscale method*. It includes modeling capillaries as one 1D channel carrying flow and particular mathematical operators used to model their interaction with the surrounding tissue. This was a virtual cancer model developed to investigate the spatiotemporal distribution of nanoconstructs in the vascular network. Iron oxide concentrations and temperature measurements of a few hypothesized treatments were generated in the virtual cancer model. This research in the future may guide the design of more efficient treatment techniques for cancer therapy. Nabil et al. [48] also worked on the same lines, particularly emphasizing modeling heat transfer and mass in MFH. Pearce et al. [49] developed a numerical model that extended the dominance of the local heat transfer BCs and provided a new approach to solve a numerical problem efficiently to make ordinary computing machinery to generate useful predictions. They developed the following model:

$$\rho_t c_t \frac{\partial \eta}{\partial t} = \nabla \cdot (k \nabla \eta) + Q_{gen} + Q_{met}, \quad Q_{gen} = \mathrm{Re}\{-\nabla \cdot S\} = (\sigma + \omega) \ddot{\varepsilon} |E|^2 + \omega \ddot{\mu} |H|^2 \qquad (2.26)$$

The collective behavior of iron oxide MNPs can improve the electromagnetic heating of particles. The results provide the basis for analysis and modeling of heating of MNPs and will improve the design of MNPs for cancer therapy, treatment planning, and experimental interpretation. Sulman and Miller [50] used PBHTM to investigate the thermal distribution developed for exciting MNPs by electromagnetic waves and metabolic processes within a spherical tumor surrounded by a sphere of healthy tissue. Their formulated models for both regions are represented by the following equations:

$$\rho_1 c_1 \frac{\partial \eta_1}{\partial t} = \frac{k_1}{r^2} \frac{\partial}{\partial r}\left(r^2 \frac{\partial \eta_1}{\partial r}\right) - c_b \omega_{b1}(\eta_1)(\eta_1 - \eta_b) + P \qquad (2.27)$$

$$\rho_2 c_2 \frac{\partial \eta_2}{\partial t} = \frac{k_2}{r^2} \frac{\partial}{\partial r}\left(r^2 \frac{\partial \eta_2}{\partial r}\right) - c_b \omega_{b2}(\eta_2)(\eta_2 - \eta_b) \qquad (2.28)$$

Numerical results for BHTM with blood perfusion were demonstrated and compared with those of the traditional PBHTM with a constant perfusion rate. Moreover, they investigated the dependence of tissue temperature and MNP heat production on the volume fraction of MNPs. In another study, Wang et al. [51] developed three models: (1) Thermo-seed thermogenesis model. (2) Tissue heat transfer model. (3) Tissue thermal damage model. These were based on the 4D energy field, thermal damage field, and temperature field distributions demonstrating. These models are represented by the following equations:

Thermo-seed Model:

$$H_z = AI_0(\beta r) + BK_0(\beta r), \quad \beta = j\omega\mu(\sigma + j\omega\mu) \tag{2.29}$$

$$\rho c \frac{\partial \eta}{\partial t} = \nabla \cdot (k\nabla\eta) + c_b\omega_b(\eta_b - \eta) + Q_m + Q_r, \quad Q_m = Q_{m0}\varphi^{\left(\frac{T-37}{10}\right)} \tag{2.30}$$

$$\Omega = A \int_0^\tau e^{-\frac{E}{RT(x, y, z, t)}} dt \tag{2.31}$$

where A is the frequency factor, R is the universal gas constant, E is the activation energy, and $T(x,y,z,t)$ is the absolute tissue temperature. Simulations were performed using the finite volume method (FVM). The reliability of the MFH model was verified using computer simulations and experimental results that were in good agreement. This research promoted the application of induction therapy, conformal hypertherapy, and enhanced the accuracy of tissue thermal damage distribution predictions and the temperature field.

2.2 Analytical modeling of MFH

Based on certain assumptions and simplifications, some researchers analytically modeled MFH. Andrä et al. [52] considered MNPs to be an exact sphere and analytically derived temperature versus time and space curves. His validation of analytical results with experimental results was in good agreement. Later, Sawyer et al. [53] confirmed this solution. Bagaria and Johnson [54] incorporated the blood perfusion rate in their analytical model for MFH. They used the method of separation of variables to solve the model taking quadratic polynomials. They also argued that higher-order polynomials are impractical. Durkee [55] analytically derived 1D solution of the bioheat transfer model while dealing with MFH. Michele et al. [56] dealt with the infusion model solution analytically with thermal excitation processes.

2.3 Numerical modeling of MFH

Numerical modeling offers solutions to those issues which cannot be dealt with costly and time-consuming experiments [57]. Based on assumptions, analytical solutions do not give accurate solutions; therefore, numerical modeling based on FEM and FDM techniques presents accurate solutions with geometrical flexibility. Sawyer et al. [53] used iron-cobalt MNPs to model MFH based on the FEM method. Their validation with Andrä et al.'s [58] results was in good agreement. Candeo and Dughiero [59] investigated the impact of MNPs of different sizes using the FEM method. Pearce et al. [60] investigated heat dissipation by different MNPs. They incorporated Fe_3O_4 MNPs in their study using FEM models of all dynamically involved equations. Pavel and Stancu [61] also applied the same technique to investigate the decrement in tumor temperature. Jeyadevan [62] predicted specific heat absorption and thermophysical properties of magnetite MNPs using a numerical modeling approach. Pavel and Stancu [63], using the FEM modeling approach, investigated the impact of a nearby blood vessels on tumor hyperthermia and also tumors of different sizes and shapes.

Paruch [64] incorporated iron oxide MNPs in artificial hyperthermia to kill tumor cells. Sawicki et al. [65] used Fe_2O_3 MNPs and the FEM method to develop a realistic model based on blood perfusion, metabolic heat, and convective heat exchange with the environment. Majchrzak and Paruch [66] used Fe_3O_4 MNPs and the Boundary Element Method (BEM) for thermal therapy of cancer. Gooneratne et al. [67] dealt with MFH with different weight densities of magnetic nanofluid. Using larger magnetoresistance (GMR) probe, these may be estimated in the tumor tissue. Pearce et al. [60] employed Fe_3O_4 MNPs and the FEM method to predict the heat generation by the MNPs that were collected and evenly dispersed. Pearce et al. [40] applied MFH to treat mouse mammary carcinoma using the FEM method and iron oxide MNPs. Reis et al. [68] dealt with CUDA with parallelization using both maghemite and magnetite MNPs. This study was based on the FDM method.

2.4 Optimization in MFH

In MFH, Optimization is effective for maximizing the therapeutic effects and minimizing the side effects. All the optimization techniques can be classified into the gradient and nongradient approaches. Many researchers applied different optimizing techniques in MFH [29]. Koch and Winfrey [57] used the Crank-Nicolson scheme to optimize the energy density in the tumor while minimizing the side effects on normal healthy tissues. They also validated their results with that of Ref. [69] in good agreement. Bagaria and Johnson [54] optimized the thermal temperature using the penalty function in MFH. Mital and Tafreshi [70] optimized the therapeutic time to be 1-h using a fitness function. Salloum et al. [29] also optimized the therapeutic time by constructing piecewise objective functions. Faktorova and Papezova [71] optimized the time for thermal therapy to be 8min based on the pharmacokinetics model. Tsuda et al. [72] optimized the electrode configuration in capacitive hyperthermia. They developed the fitness function using the inversion method based on the 2D-FEM solution of the Laplace equation. Mital and Tafreshi [70] optimized the thermal damage in MFH using the Genetic algorithm (GA). Loulou and Scott [58] applied the conjugate gradient method in the optimization of hyperthermia processes. Paolo di Barab et al. [73] optimized the distribution of MNPs in the tumor using GA.

Mario Wolf et al. [74] optimized the heat supply using the Steepest Descent Method (SDM). Guanzhong Hu et al. [75] optimized the temperature field using Particle Swarm Optimization (PSO) and the Multiobjective Algorithm. Lalonde and Hunt [76] optimized ultrasound focused distribution using the Simplex Algorithm. Syed Hassan and Jungwon Yoon [77] optimized a real-time targeted drug delivery system using PSO. Rodrigues [69] applied both the experimental and numerical approaches to optimize the virtual human chest model. Manu Mital [70] optimized the thermal damage of the tumor using the Gradient Algorithm. Phong Thanh Nguyen [78] optimized the antenna design using PSO. Phong Thanh Nguyen et al. [10] used the same method to optimize amplitude and phase excitations of antenna elements.

2.5 Integrated therapies

MFH in integration with chemotherapy and radiation therapies produces more productive results [79]. Integrating with radiation gives fast tumor damage [80,81]. MFH's integration with other therapies is shown in Fig. 2.1. A higher thermal enhancement ratio can be achieved

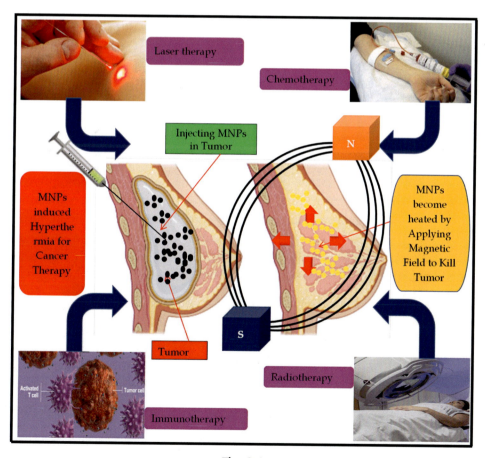

Fig. 2.1
Integration of MFH with chemotherapy, laser therapy, radiotherapy, or immunotherapy treatment modalities.

using therapies in integration [82], which is the ratio of sensitivity at some elevated temperature to the sensitivity at 37.5°C [83]. The literature shows that heat can be combined with radiation [84,85] and derivation of heating time and applications of algorithm are also crucial [86]. In vivo studies show that the survival rates of animals increase when combined treatment is used [87]. Ito et al. [88] combined immunotherapy with MFH to treat murine melanoma B16 with positive results.

Terentyuk [89] used photothermal therapy in integration with plasmonic silica/gold nanoshell-induced hyperthermia for successful therapy. Guibert et al. [90] used dynamic light scattering (DLS) with MFH for effective heating efficiency. Jiang et al. [91] used radiotherapy with MFH to treat the tumor with promising results. Petryk et al. [92] combined microwave hypertherapy and MFH to eradicate the mouse mammary adenocarcinoma in the clinical setting. Sturesson and Andersson Engels [93] worked a combined therapy of laser and MFH for the bovine liver model. Cheng et al. [94] integrated infrared photothermal therapy with MFH for tumor eradication. Xu et al. [95] integrated laser therapy with MFH for thermal therapy of cancerous tissue. Quinto et al. [96] combined MFH with Radiotherapy and Chemotherapy for effective tumor regression.

2.6 In vivo experimental studies of MFH

One of the major challenges for in vivo studies of MFH is the deficiency of colloidal stability. To tackle this issue, liposomes with MNPs of size 10nm are combined with drug delivery tools that are used in MFH. When magnetite cationic liposomes (MCLs) are administered in the tumor, its temperature is elevated above 43°C. It produced complete eradication of mammary carcinomas as a result of hyperthermia [97]. Jimbow et al. [98] used magnetite particle (NPrCAP/M)-induced MFH to treat mouse melanoma. Gordon et al. [21] treated cancers in mouse, human prostate, rate glioma, mice melanoma, carcinomas in rabbit tongue, and nude mice breast cancer using MFH and reported complete tumor eradication.

Balivada et al. [99] applied core-shell MNPs to treat mice melanoma by varying AMF exposure after every 10min. Zhao et al. [100] applied MFH to treat head and neck cancer. Verde et al. [101] used cobalt-ferrite MNPs to investigate the impact of magnetic anisotropy on the SAR where SAR was taken as a function of saturation magnetization, magnetic anisotropy, particle size, and coercive field. Suto et al. [102] investigated the impact of relaxation constants on the heat generation by MNPs. They showed that using MNPs of size 12nm through Neel relaxation gave good validation with theoretical results. Jordan et al. [103] used MFH to treat malignant brain tumors.

Yanase et al. [104] applied MFH to treat solid glioma of female F344 rats and thermal therapy gave complete tumor regression of group IV rats. Kennedy et al. [105] reviewed in detail the

MFH of in vivo studies using Gold MNPs. Salloum et al. [106] studied MFH on rat hind limbs with special emphasis on the blood perfusion rate. Kabashin et al. [107] treated lung carcinoma using Si MNP MFH. Nikolai et al. [108] successfully eradicated whole mouse tumor using MFH. Elsherbini et al. [109] treated female mice carcinoma using iron oxide Fe_3O_4 MNP-induced MFH. They used radiofrequency at 25 kW for 20 min and the temperature was elevated to 47±1°C. Shinkai et al. [110] treated the solid glioma of F344 rats using MFH. Three successive heat dosages were applied and the tumor was completely removed from the rats.

2.7 In vitro experimental studies on MFH

Johannsen et al. [111] treated the prostate cancer of a 67-year-old man with MNPs coated with amino saline. Using AMF of 100 kHz, the temperature of the tumor was elevated to 48.5–40.0°C for the first treatment and 42.5–39.4°C for the next treatment. In another work, Johannsen et al. [112] treated 10 patients with prostate cancer using MFH where the maximum temperature was elevated to 55°C. Later, they treated 22 patients with different cancers such as sarcoma, prostate, ovarian, rectal, and cervix cancers. At the end of the experiment, all the mice died and those MNPs gathered in the liver were extracted from the body by natural process [112–114].

Toshiaki Saida [97] with his team completely removed the 7-cm neck cancer at the Cancer Treatment Center of Tobata Kyouritsu Hospital through successive applications of MFH. Maier-Hauff et al. [115] treated glioblastomas using 5-mL magnetite (Fe_3O_4) MNP (12 nm)-induced MFH with promising results. Silva [116] reviewed in detail the in vitro for MFH of gliomas. Johannsen et al. [117] discussed the clinical applications of MFH in prostate cancers. They urged to the use of MFH in combination with other therapies for better treatment results. Johannsen et al. [118] treated prostate carcinoma with six successive treatments on a weekly basis, each having a 1-h duration, and got productive results. Mahmoudi and Hadjipanayis [119] treated brain tumors successfully using iron oxide MNP-induced MFH.

2.8 Case study on MFH

In a case study [120], the MFH was applied to intramuscularly implanted mammary carcinoma in a mouse. A nonaveraged volume approach based on the logistic operation was applied for each therapeutic modality. All implanted tumors were randomized 1 month after transplantation. The overall size distribution ranges from 120 to 400 mm^3. A temperature of 47°C was maintained for half an hour under the influence of an external magnetic field with an amplitude of 6–12.5 kA/m at 520 kHz. The MNPs were high biocompatible, dextran magnetite. A widespread tumor necrosis was observed. Tumor growth was slightly delayed in comparison with untreated controls. The regression analysis of MFH data yielded a smaller tumor volume of 1000 mm^3 after 50 days.

References

[1] Patterson J, Strang R. The role of blood flow in hyperthermia. Int J Radiat Oncol Biol Phys 1979;5:235–41.
[2] Miaskowski A, Sawicki B. Magnetic fluid hyperthermia modeling based on phantom measurements and realistic breast model. IEEE Trans Biomed Eng 2013;60:1806–13.
[3] Pennes HH. Analysis of tissue and arterial blood temperatures in the resting human forearm. J Appl Physiol 1948;1:93–122.
[4] Wulff W. The energy conservation equation for living tissue. IEEE Trans Biomed Eng 1974;494–5.
[5] Chen MM, Holmes KR. Microvascular contributions in tissue heat transfer. Ann N Y Acad Sci 1980;335:137–50.
[6] Jiji L, Weinbaum S, Lemons D. Theory and experiment for the effect of vascular microstructure on surface tissue heat transfer—part II: model formulation and solution. J Biomech Eng 1984;106:331–41.
[7] Weinbaum S, Jiji L. A new simplified bioheat equation for the effect of blood flow on local average tissue temperature. J Biomech Eng 1985;107:131–9.
[8] Balidemaj E, Kok HP, Schooneveldt G, van Lier AL, Remis RF, Stalpers LJ, et al. Hyperthermia treatment planning for cervical cancer patients based on electrical conductivity tissue properties acquired in vivo with EPT at 3 T MRI. Int J Hyperth 2016;32:558–68.
[9] Deuflhard P, Seebass M, Stalling D, Beck R, Hege H-C. Hyperthermia treatment planning in clinical cancer therapy: modelling, simulation and visualization; 1997.
[10] Nguyen PT, Abbosh A, Crozier S. Three-dimensional microwave hyperthermia for breast cancer treatment in a realistic environment using particle swarm optimization. IEEE Trans Biomed Eng 2017;64:1335–44.
[11] Arkin H, Xu L, Holmes K. Recent developments in modeling heat transfer in blood perfused tissues. IEEE Trans Biomed Eng 1994;41:97–107.
[12] Baish J, Ayyaswamy P, Foster K. Heat transport mechanisms in vascular tissues: a model comparison. J Biomech Eng 1986;108:324–31.
[13] Charny C, Levin R. Bioheat transfer in a branching countercurrent network during hyperthermia. J Biomech Eng 1989;111:263–70.
[14] Wissler E. Comments on the new bioheat equation proposed by Weinbaum and Jiji. J Biomech Eng 1987;109:226.
[15] Jamil M, Ng EY-K. To optimize the efficacy of bioheat transfer in capacitive hyperthermia: a physical perspective. J Therm Biol 2013;38:272–9.
[16] Tzou D. Transfer M-tMH. Washington, DC: Taylor & Francis; 1997. p. 138–46.
[17] Rubio MFJC, Hernández AV, Salas LL. High temperature hyperthermia in breast cancer treatment. In: Hyperthermia. IntechOpen; 2013.
[18] Majchrzak E, Turchan Ł. Numerical analysis of tissue heating using the bioheat transfer porous model. Comput Assisted Methods Eng Sci 2017;20:123–31.
[19] Gilchrist R, Medal R, Shorey WD, Hanselman RC, Parrott JC, Taylor CB. Selective inductive heating of lymph nodes. Ann Surg 1957;146:596.
[20] Kobayashi T, Kakimi K, Nakayama E, Jimbow K. Antitumor immunity by magnetic nanoparticle-mediated hyperthermia. Nanomedicine 2014;9:1715–26.
[21] Gordon R, Hines J, Gordon D. Intracellular hyperthermia a biophysical approach to cancer treatment via intracellular temperature and biophysical alterations. Med Hypotheses 1979;5:83–102.
[22] LeBrun A, Manuchehrabadi N, Attaluri A, Wang F, Ma R, Zhu L. MicroCT image-generated tumour geometry and SAR distribution for tumour temperature elevation simulations in magnetic nanoparticle hyperthermia. Int J Hyperth 2013;29:730–8.
[23] LeBrun A, Ma R, Zhu L. MicroCT image based simulation to design heating protocols in magnetic nanoparticle hyperthermia for cancer treatment. J Therm Biol 2016;62:129–37.
[24] Eagle S, Wadsworth S, Wnorowski A. Modeling an injection profile of nanoparticles to optimize tumor treatment time with magnetic hyperthermia; 2015.
[25] Sankar S, Zhang M. Optimization of combined radiation and gold nanoparticle hyperthermia therapy for treating cutaneous squamous carcinoma; 2015.

[26] Hainfeld JF, Lin L, Slatkin DN, Dilmanian FA, Vadas TM, Smilowitz HM. Gold nanoparticle hyperthermia reduces radiotherapy dose. Nanomedicine 2014;10:1609–17.

[27] Kim B, Han G, Toley BJ, Kim C-k, Rotello VM, Forbes NS. Tuning payload delivery in tumour cylindroids using gold nanoparticles. Nat Nanotechnol 2010;5:465.

[28] Javidi M, Heydari M, Karimi A, Haghpanahi M, Navidbakhsh M, Razmkon A. Evaluation of the effects of injection velocity and different gel concentrations on nanoparticles in hyperthermia therapy. J Biomed Phys Eng 2014;4:151.

[29] Salloum M, Ma R, Zhu L. Enhancement in treatment planning for magnetic nanoparticle hyperthermia: optimization of the heat absorption pattern. Int J Hyperth 2009;25:309–21.

[30] Hall M, Yanga D, Yi K, Zhou J. Optimized injection site location for magnetic nanoparticle induced hyperthermia cancer treatment; 2012.

[31] Perigo EA, Hemery G, Sandre O, Ortega D, Garaio E, Plazaola F, et al. Fundamentals and advances in magnetic hyperthermia. Appl Phys Rev 2015;2, 041302.

[32] Liangruksa M, Ganguly R, Puri IK. Parametric investigation of heating due to magnetic fluid hyperthermia in a tumor with blood perfusion. J Magn Magn Mater 2011;323:708–16.

[33] Maenosono S, Saita S. Theoretical assessment of FePt nanoparticles as heating elements for magnetic hyperthermia. IEEE Trans Magn 2006;42:1638–42.

[34] Liu K-C, Chen H-T. Analysis for the dual-phase-lag bio-heat transfer during magnetic hyperthermia treatment. Int J Heat Mass Transf 2009;52:1185–92.

[35] Wu J, Ma X, Wang Y. Hyperthermia cancer therapy by magnetic nanoparticles; 2013.

[36] Branquinho LC, Carrião MS, Costa AS, Zufelato N, Sousa MH, Miotto R, et al. Effect of magnetic dipolar interactions on nanoparticle heating efficiency: implications for cancer hyperthermia. Sci Rep 2013;3:2887.

[37] Rast L, Harrison JG. Computational modeling of electromagnetically induced heating of magnetic nanoparticle materials for hyperthermic cancer treatment. PIERS Online 2010;6:690–4.

[38] Feng Y, Rylander M, Bass J, Oden J, Diller K. Optimal design of laser surgery for cancer treatment through nanoparticle-mediated hyperthermia therapy. In: NSTI-Nanotech2005; 2005. p. 39–42.

[39] Bellizzi G, Bucci OM, Chirico G. Numerical assessment of a criterion for the optimal choice of the operative conditions in magnetic nanoparticle hyperthermia on a realistic model of the human head. Int J Hyperth 2016;32:688–703.

[40] Pearce JA, Petyk AA, Hoopes PJ. FEM numerical model analysis of magnetic nanoparticle tumor heating experiments. In: 2014 36th annual international conference of the IEEE Engineering in Medicine and Biology Society. IEEE; 2014. p. 5312–5.

[41] Bhowmick S, Coad J, Swanlund D, Bischof J. In vitro thermal therapy of AT-1 dunning prostate tumours. Int J Hyperth 2004;20:73–92.

[42] Huang H-C, Rege K, Heys JJ. Spatiotemporal temperature distribution and cancer cell death in response to extracellular hyperthermia induced by gold nanorods. ACS Nano 2010;4:2892–900.

[43] Moritz AR, Henriques Jr F. Studies of thermal injury: II. The relative importance of time and surface temperature in the causation of cutaneous burns. Am J Pathol 1947;23:695.

[44] Elliott A, Schwartz J, Wang J, Shetty A, Hazle J, Stafford JR. Analytical solution to heat equation with magnetic resonance experimental verification for nanoshell enhanced thermal therapy. Lasers Surg Med 2008;40:660–5.

[45] Huang X, Jain PK, El-Sayed IH, El-Sayed MA. Determination of the minimum temperature required for selective photothermal destruction of cancer cells with the use of immunotargeted gold nanoparticles. Photochem Photobiol 2006;82:412–7.

[46] Xu R, Zhang Y, Ma M, Xia J, Liu J, Guo Q, et al. Measurement of specific absorption rate and thermal simulation for arterial embolization hyperthermia in the maghemite-gelled model. IEEE Trans Magn 2007;43:1078–85.

[47] Nabil M, Zunino P. A computational study of cancer hyperthermia based on vascular magnetic nanoconstructs. R Soc Open Sci 2016;3, 160287.

[48] Nabil M, Decuzzi P, Zunino P. Modelling mass and heat transfer in nano-based cancer hyperthermia. R Soc Open Sci 2015;2, 150447.

[49] Pearce J, Giustini A, Stigliano R, Hoopes PJ. Magnetic heating of nanoparticles: the importance of particle clustering to achieve therapeutic temperatures. J Nanotechnol Eng Med 2013;4, 011005.

[50] Sulman MM, Miller DF, Kozlowski G. Nonlinear model for magnetic nanoparticle-based hyperthermia. Int J Math Model Numer Optim 2015;6:223–34.

[51] Wang H, Wu J, Zhuo Z, Tang J. A three-dimensional model and numerical simulation regarding thermoseed mediated magnetic induction therapy conformal hyperthermia. Technol Health Care 2016;24:S827–39.

[52] Andrä W, d'Ambly C, Hergt R, Hilger I, Kaiser W. Temperature distribution as function of time around a small spherical heat source of local magnetic hyperthermia. J Magn Magn Mater 1999;194:197–203.

[53] Sawyer CA, Habib AH, Miller K, Collier KN, Ondeck CL, McHenry ME. Modeling of temperature profile during magnetic thermotherapy for cancer treatment. J Appl Phys 2009;105:07B320.

[54] Bagaria H, Johnson D. Transient solution to the bioheat equation and optimization for magnetic fluid hyperthermia treatment. Int J Hyperth 2005;21:57–75.

[55] Durkee Jr J, Antich P, Lee C. Exact solutions to the multiregion time-dependent bioheat equation. I: solution development. Phys Med Biol 1990;35:847.

[56] Di Michele F, Pizzichelli G, Mazzolai B, Sinibaldi E. On the preliminary design of hyperthermia treatments based on infusion and heating of magnetic nanofluids. Math Biosci 2015;262:105–16.

[57] Koch CM, Winfrey AL. FEM optimization of energy density in tumor hyperthermia using time-dependent magnetic nanoparticle power dissipation. IEEE Trans Magn 2014;50:1–7.

[58] Loulou T, Scott EP. Thermal dose optimization in hyperthermia treatments by using the conjugate gradient method. Numer Heat Transfer Part A 2002;42:661–83.

[59] Candeo A, Dughiero F. Numerical FEM models for the planning of magnetic induction hyperthermia treatments with nanoparticles. IEEE Trans Magn 2009;45:1658–61.

[60] Pearce JA, Cook JR, Hoopes PJ, Giustini A. FEM numerical model study of heating in magnetic nanoparticles. In: Energy-based treatment of tissue and assessment VI. International Society for Optics and Photonics; 2011. p. 79010B.

[61] Pavel M, Stancu A. Ferromagnetic nanoparticles dose based on tumor size in magnetic fluid hyperthermia cancer therapy. IEEE Trans Magn 2009;45:5251–4.

[62] Jeyadevan B. Present status and prospects of magnetite nanoparticles-based hyperthermia. J Ceram Soc Jpn 2010;118:391–401.

[63] Pavel M, Stancu A. Study of the optimum injection sites for a multiple metastases region in cancer therapy by using MFH. IEEE Trans Magn 2009;45:4825–8.

[64] Paruch M. Hyperthermia process control induced by the electric field in order to cancer destroying. Acta Bioeng Biomech 2014;16:123–30.

[65] Sawicki B, Miaskowski A. Numerical model of magnetic fluid hyperthermia. Prz Elektrotech 2013;89:86–8.

[66] Majchrzak E, Paruch M. Numerical modelling of the cancer destruction during hyperthermia treatment. In: 19th international conference on computer methods in mechanics CMM-2011, Warsaw, Poland, short papers; 2001. p. 333–4.

[67] Gooneratne CP, Kurnicki A, Yamada S, Mukhopadhyay SC, Kosel J. Analysis of the distribution of magnetic fluid inside tumors by a giant magnetoresistance probe. PLoS One 2013;8, e81227.

[68] Reis RF, dos Santos Loureiro F, Lobosco M. 3D numerical simulations on GPUs of hyperthermia with nanoparticles by a nonlinear bioheat model. J Comput Appl Math 2016;295:35–47.

[69] Rodrigues DB, Hurwitz MD, Maccarini PF, Stauffer PR. Optimization of chest wall hyperthermia treatment using a virtual human chest model. In: 2015 9th European conference on antennas and propagation (EuCAP). IEEE; 2015. p. 1–5.

[70] Mital M, Tafreshi HV. A methodology for determining optimal thermal damage in magnetic nanoparticle hyperthermia cancer treatment. Int J Numer Methods Biomed Eng 2012;28:205–13.

[71] Faktorová D, Pápežová M. Optimization of mild microwave hyperthermia interconnection with targeted delivery of nanoparticles. Prz Elektrotech 2014;90:117–9.

[72] Tsuda N, Kuroda K, Suzuki Y. An inverse method to optimize heating conditions in RF-capacitive hyperthermia. IEEE Trans Biomed Eng 1996;43:1029–37.

[73] Di Barba P, Dughiero F, Sieni E. Field synthesis for the optimal treatment planning in magnetic fluid hyperthermia. Arch Electr Eng 2012;61:57–67.

[74] Wolf M, Rath K, Ruiz AER, Kühnicke E. Ultrasound thermometry for optimizing heat supply during a hyperthermia therapy of cancer tissue. Phys Procedia 2015;70:888–91.

[75] Hu G, Li Y, Yang S, Bai Y, Huang J. Temperature field optimization and magnetic nanoparticles optimal approximation of MFH for cancer therapy. IEEE Trans Magn 2015;51:1–4.

[76] Lalonde RJ, Hunt JW. Optimizing ultrasound focus distributions for hyperthermia. IEEE Trans Biomed Eng 1995;42:981–90.

[77] Hassan S, Yoon J. Nano carriers based targeted drug delivery path planning using hybrid particle swarm optimizer and artificial magnetic fields. In: 2012 12th international conference on control, automation and systems. IEEE; 2012. p. 1700–5.

[78] Nguyen PT. Focusing microwave hyperthermia in realistic environment for breast cancer treatment [PhD thesis]. University of Queensland; 2015.

[79] Datta N, Krishnan S, Speiser D, Neufeld E, Kuster N, Bodis S, et al. Magnetic nanoparticle-induced hyperthermia with appropriate payloads: Paul Ehrlich's "magic (nano) bullet" for cancer theranostics? Cancer Treat Rev 2016;50:217–27.

[80] Dewhirst M. Thermal dosimetry: thermo-radiotherapy and thermochemotherapy. Berlin: Springer-Verlag; 1995.

[81] Klemmer T, Hoydick D, Okumura H, Zhang B, Soffa W. Magnetic hardening and coercivity mechanisms in L10 ordered FePd ferromagnets. Scr Metall Mater 1995;33:1793–805.

[82] Pankhurst Q, Thanh N, Jones S, Dobson J. Progress in applications of magnetic nanoparticles in biomedicine. J Phys D Appl Phys 2009;42, 224001.

[83] Pankhurst QA, Connolly J, Jones S, Dobson J. Applications of magnetic nanoparticles in biomedicine. J Phys D Appl Phys 2003;36:R167.

[84] Inomata K, Sawa T, Hashimoto S. Effect of large boron additions to magnetically hard Fe-Pt alloys. J Appl Phys 1988;64:2537–40.

[85] Fortin J-P, Wilhelm C, Servais J, Ménager C, Bacri J-C, Gazeau F. Size-sorted anionic iron oxide nanomagnets as colloidal mediators for magnetic hyperthermia. J Am Chem Soc 2007;129:2628–35.

[86] Vassiliou JK, Mehrotra V, Russell MW, Giannelis EP, McMichael R, Shull R, et al. Magnetic and optical properties of γ-Fe2O3 nanocrystals. J Appl Phys 1993;73:5109–16.

[87] Sato T, Iijima T, Seki M, Inagaki N. Magnetic properties of ultrafine ferrite particles. J Magn Magn Mater 1987;65:252–6.

[88] Ito A, Tanaka K, Kondo K, Shinkai M, Honda H, Matsumoto K, et al. Tumor regression by combined immunotherapy and hyperthermia using magnetic nanoparticles in an experimental subcutaneous murine melanoma. Cancer Sci 2003;94:308–13.

[89] Terentyuk GS, Maslyakova GN, Suleymanova LV, Khlebtsov NG, Khlebtsov BN, Akchurin GG, et al. Laser-induced tissue hyperthermia mediated by gold nanoparticles: toward cancer phototherapy. J Biomed Opt 2009;14, 021016.

[90] Guibert C, Dupuis V, Peyre V, Fresnais J. Hyperthermia of magnetic nanoparticles: experimental study of the role of aggregation. J Phys Chem C 2015;119:28148–54.

[91] Jiang P-S, Tsai H-Y, Drake P, Wang F-N, Chiang C-S. Gadolinium-doped iron oxide nanoparticles induced magnetic field hyperthermia combined with radiotherapy increases tumour response by vascular disruption and improved oxygenation. Int J Hyperth 2017;33:770–8.

[92] Petryk AA, Giustini AJ, Gottesman RE, Trembly BS, Hoopes PJ. Comparison of magnetic nanoparticle and microwave hyperthermia cancer treatment methodology and treatment effect in a rodent breast cancer model. Int J Hyperth 2013;29:819–27.

[93] Sturesson C, Andersson-Engels S. A mathematical model for predicting the temperature distribution in laser-induced hyperthermia. Experimental evaluation and applications. Phys Med Biol 1995;40:2037.

[94] Cheng L, Yang K, Chen Q, Liu Z. Organic stealth nanoparticles for highly effective in vivo near-infrared photothermal therapy of cancer. ACS Nano 2012;6:5605–13.

[95] Xu X, Meade A, Bayazitoglu Y. Numerical investigation of nanoparticle-assisted laser-induced interstitial thermotherapy toward tumor and cancer treatments. Lasers Med Sci 2011;26:213–22.
[96] Quinto CA, Mohindra P, Tong S, Bao G. Multifunctional superparamagnetic iron oxide nanoparticles for combined chemotherapy and hyperthermia cancer treatment. Nanoscale 2015;7:12728–36.
[97] Kobayashi T. Cancer hyperthermia using magnetic nanoparticles. Biotechnol J 2011;6:1342–7.
[98] Jimbow K, Takada T, Sato M, Sato A, Kamiya T, Ono I, et al. Keynote-4 melanin biology and translational research strategy: melanogenesis and nanomedicine as the basis for melanoma-targeted Dds and chemo-thermo-immunotherapy. Pigment Cell Melanoma Res 2008;21:243–4.
[99] Balivada S, Rachakatla RS, Wang H, Samarakoon TN, Dani RK, Pyle M, et al. A/C magnetic hyperthermia of melanoma mediated by iron (0)/iron oxide core/shell magnetic nanoparticles: a mouse study. BMC Cancer 2010;10:119.
[100] Zhao Q, Wang L, Cheng R, Mao L, Arnold RD, Howerth EW, et al. Magnetic nanoparticle-based hyperthermia for head & neck cancer in mouse models. Theranostics 2012;2:113.
[101] Verde EL, Landi GT, Gomes JA, Sousa MH, Bakuzis AF. Magnetic hyperthermia investigation of cobalt ferrite nanoparticles: comparison between experiment, linear response theory, and dynamic hysteresis simulations. J Appl Phys 2012;111, 123902.
[102] Suto M, Hirota Y, Mamiya H, Fujita A, Kasuya R, Tohji K, et al. Heat dissipation mechanism of magnetite nanoparticles in magnetic fluid hyperthermia. J Magn Magn Mater 2009;321:1493–6.
[103] Jordan A, Scholz R, Maier-Hauff K, van Landeghem FK, Waldoefner N, Teichgraeber U, et al. The effect of thermotherapy using magnetic nanoparticles on rat malignant glioma. J Neuro-Oncol 2006;78:7–14.
[104] Yanase M, Shinkai M, Honda H, Wakabayashi T, Yoshida J, Kobayashi T. Intracellular hyperthermia for cancer using magnetite cationic liposomes: an in vivo study. Jpn J Cancer Res 1998;89:463–70.
[105] Kennedy LC, Bickford LR, Lewinski NA, Coughlin AJ, Hu Y, Day ES, et al. A new era for cancer treatment: gold-nanoparticle-mediated thermal therapies. Small 2011;7:169–83.
[106] Salloum M, Ma R, Zhu L. An in-vivo experimental study of temperature elevations in animal tissue during magnetic nanoparticle hyperthermia. Int J Hyperth 2008;24:589–601.
[107] Kabashin A, Tamarov K, Ryabchikov YV, Osminkina L, Zinovyev S, Kargina J, et al. Si nanoparticles as sensitizers for radio frequency-induced cancer hyperthermia. In: Synthesis and photonics of nanoscale materials XIII. International Society for Optics and Photonics; 2016. p. 97370A.
[108] Brusentsov NA, Nikitin LV, Brusentsova TN, Kuznetsov AA, Bayburtskiy FS, Shumakov LI, et al. Magnetic fluid hyperthermia of the mouse experimental tumor. J Magn Magn Mater 2002;252:378–80.
[109] Elsherbini AA, Saber M, Aggag M, El-Shahawy A, Shokier HA. Magnetic nanoparticle-induced hyperthermia treatment under magnetic resonance imaging. Magn Reson Imaging 2011;29:272–80.
[110] Shinkai M, Yanase M, Suzuki M, Honda H, Wakabayashi T, Yoshida J, et al. Intracellular hyperthermia for cancer using magnetite cationic liposomes. J Magn Magn Mater 1999;194:176–84.
[111] Johannsen M, Gneveckow U, Eckelt L, Feussner A, Waldöfner N, Scholz R, et al. Clinical hyperthermia of prostate cancer using magnetic nanoparticles: presentation of a new interstitial technique. Int J Hyperth 2005;21:637–47.
[112] Johannsen M, Gneveckow U, Taymoorian K, Thiesen B, Waldöfner N, Scholz R, et al. Morbidity and quality of life during thermotherapy using magnetic nanoparticles in locally recurrent prostate cancer: results of a prospective phase I trial. Int J Hyperth 2007;23:315–23.
[113] Wust P, Gneveckow U, Wust P, Gneveckow U, Johannsen M, Böhmer D, et al. Magnetic nanoparticles for interstitial thermotherapy–feasibility, tolerance and achieved temperatures. Int J Hyperth 2006;22:673–85.
[114] Ito A, Nakahara Y, Tanaka K, Kuga Y, Honda H, Kobayashi T. Time course of biodistribution and heat generation of magnetite cationic liposomes in mouse model. Therm Med 2003;19:151–9.
[115] Maier-Hauff K, Ulrich F, Nestler D, Niehoff H, Wust P, Thiesen B, et al. Efficacy and safety of intratumoral thermotherapy using magnetic iron-oxide nanoparticles combined with external beam radiotherapy on patients with recurrent glioblastoma multiforme. J Neuro-Oncol 2011;103:317–24.
[116] Silva AC, Oliveira TR, Mamani JB, Malheiros SM, Malavolta L, Pavon LF, et al. Application of hyperthermia induced by superparamagnetic iron oxide nanoparticles in glioma treatment. Int J Nanomedicine 2011;6:591.

[117] Johannsen M, Thiesen B, Wust P, Jordan A. Magnetic nanoparticle hyperthermia for prostate cancer. Int J Hyperth 2010;26:790–5.
[118] Johannsen M, Gneveckow U, Eckelt L, Feussner A, Waldoefner N, Scholz R, et al. Clinical hyperthermia of prostate cancer using magnetic nanoparticles-preliminary experience with a new interstitial technique. Int J Hyperth 2005;21:637–47.
[119] Mahmoudi K, Hadjipanayis CG. The application of magnetic nanoparticles for the treatment of brain tumors. Front Chem 2014;2:109.
[120] Jordan A, Scholz R, Wust P, Fähling H, Krause J, Wlodarczyk W, et al. Effects of magnetic fluid hyperthermia (MFH) on C3H mammary carcinoma in vivo. Int J Hyperth 1997;13:587–605.

CHAPTER 3

The phenomena of heat dissipation by magnetic nanoparticles under applied magnetic field

3.1 The force acting on nanoparticles under an applied magnetic field

The force acting on spherical MNPs under the magnetic field [1,2] is given by

$$\mathbf{F}_m = (\mathbf{m} \cdot \nabla)\mathbf{B} \tag{3.1}$$

where **m** is the magnetic moment of MNP, which depends on the material and volume of the MNPs, and $\mathbf{B}$ is an external magnetic field. For an MNP suspended in a fluid, the total magnetic moment can be expressed as

$$\mathbf{m} = V_m \mathbf{M} \tag{3.2}$$

where V_m is the volume of MNPs and $\mathbf{M}$ is the volumetric magnetization and is expressed as

$$\mathbf{M} = \Delta\chi \mathbf{H} \tag{3.3}$$

where $\Delta\chi = \chi_m - \chi_f$ is the relative susceptibility of MNPs in the fluid. The overall response of MNPs and fluid is expressed as

$$\mathbf{B} = \mu_0 \mathbf{H} \tag{3.4}$$

With this, the magnetic force becomes

$$\mathbf{F}_m = \frac{V_m \Delta\chi}{\mu_0}(\mathbf{B} \cdot \nabla)\mathbf{B} \tag{3.5}$$

3.2 Maxwell's equations of electromagnetism

The interaction of the electromagnetic field with the human body can be understood through Maxwell's equations [3,4]. For the given magnetic field source, Maxwell equations can be solved in a closed-form solution subjected to boundary conditions [5]. The electric field, E, is the sum of the electric field, E_q, present due to electric charges and electric field, E_m, due to time-dependent magnetic flux density, $\varepsilon = \varepsilon_r \varepsilon_0$. The electric flux density, **D**, in a dielectric medium with dielectric permeability, ε_r, is defined as

$$\boldsymbol{B} = \nabla \times \boldsymbol{A} \tag{3.6}$$

where ε and ε_0 are the dielectric constant of medium and free space, respectively. The electric field gives rise to the magnetic field **H** through Ampere's Law with path length l and current **I**.

$$\oint_l \boldsymbol{H} \cdot t\, dl = \boldsymbol{I} \tag{3.7}$$

Under the quasistatic hypothesis, Maxwell equations are defined as

$$\nabla \cdot \boldsymbol{D} = \rho \tag{3.8}$$

$$\nabla \cdot \boldsymbol{B} = 0 \tag{3.9}$$

$$\nabla \times \boldsymbol{E} = -\frac{\partial \boldsymbol{B}}{\partial t} \tag{3.10}$$

$$\nabla \times \boldsymbol{H} = \boldsymbol{J} + \frac{\partial \boldsymbol{D}}{\partial t} \tag{3.11}$$

where ρ is the volume charge density, μ is the magnetic permeability of the medium, and $\mu = \mu_r \mu_0$ where μ_r and μ_0 are the relative permeability of medium and vacuum, respectively. The magnetic and electric flux densities are correlated with magnetic and electric fields, respectively, as

$$\boldsymbol{D} = \varepsilon \boldsymbol{E} \tag{3.12}$$

$$\boldsymbol{B} = \mu \boldsymbol{H} \tag{3.13}$$

$$\boldsymbol{J} = \sigma \boldsymbol{E} \tag{3.14}$$

3.3 The magnetic vector potential

The magnetic field, **B**, being solenoid is related to the magnetic vector potential as

$$\boldsymbol{B} = \nabla \times \boldsymbol{A} \tag{3.15}$$

Substituting the above equation in Eq. (3.10):

$$\nabla \times \boldsymbol{E} = -\frac{\partial \boldsymbol{B}}{\partial t} = -\frac{\partial (\nabla \times \boldsymbol{A})}{\partial t} \Rightarrow -\nabla \times \left(\boldsymbol{E} + \frac{\partial \boldsymbol{A}}{\partial t}\right) = 0 \tag{3.16}$$

3.4 The scalar electric potential

For the irrotational field, the scalar electric potential is related to vector magnetic potential as

$$-\nabla V = E + \frac{\partial A}{\partial t} \tag{3.17}$$

And the electric field can be calculated as

$$E = -\left(\nabla V + \frac{\partial A}{\partial t}\right) \tag{3.18}$$

The current density, J, being solenoidal can be demonstrated as a curl of the electric vector potential [6–9],

$$J = \nabla \times T \tag{3.19}$$

The magnetic vector potential, Φ, can be defined analogously to an electric field,

$$\nabla \times H = J = \nabla \times T \Rightarrow \nabla \times (H - T) = 0 \tag{3.20}$$

The scalar magnetic potential in a gradient form can be defined as

$$-\nabla \Phi = H - T \tag{3.21}$$

Writing H as a difference of T and gradient of Φ,

$$H = T - \nabla \Phi \tag{3.22}$$

3.5 Hysteresis curve and coercivity

Heat in MNPs can be generated through Neel relaxation, Brownian relaxation, photothermal effect, or hysteresis loss by the application of AMF. Heat in bulk materials is generated by Eddy currents and does not apply to MNPs because of low electrical conductivity and hysteresis loss is favorable for macroparticles. The coercivity on particle volume can be represented as

$$H_c = \left(\frac{2K}{M_s}\right)\left[1 - \sqrt{\frac{V_c}{V}}\right], \quad V > V_c \tag{3.23}$$

where V_c represents the critical volume. The relaxation effects appear below this limit. The major cause of heat generation in MNPs is the rotation of magnetic moments opposite to the energy barrier. For applied AMF, magnetization follows the hysteresis loop, which is addressed by saturation magnetization (M_s), coercivity (H_c), and remnant magnetization (M_r), as demonstrated in Fig. 3.1. The closed hysteresis loop area represents the magnitude of total heat released [10,11].

3.6 Neel and Brownian relaxation

The Brownian relaxation effect appears when MNP itself rotates and heat is dissipated as a result of shear stress. When the particles are fixed and the moment rotates then it is acted upon

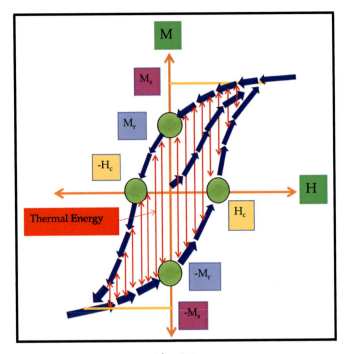

Fig. 3.1
The heat released by hysteresis loop.

by a Neel relaxational effect and energy is generated as a result of the atomic dipole moment as shown in Fig. 3.2. The Neel relaxation time is very short and was proposed by Néel [12] and after this Brown [13] modified it to the following form:

$$\tau_N = \frac{\tau_0}{2}\sqrt{\pi\left(\frac{kT}{KV_m}\right)}e^{\left(\frac{KV_m}{kT}\right)} \tag{3.24}$$

here, V and K represent the volume of the particle and anisotropy constant, respectively. Brownian relaxation time is given by

$$\tau_B = \frac{3\eta V_H}{k_B T} \tag{3.25}$$

here, V_H is the particle's hydrodynamic volume and η represents the viscosity of the nanofluid. Neel and Brownian time relaxations occur in parallel and are represented as [14]

$$\frac{1}{\tau} = \frac{1}{\tau_N} + \frac{1}{\tau_B} \tag{3.26}$$

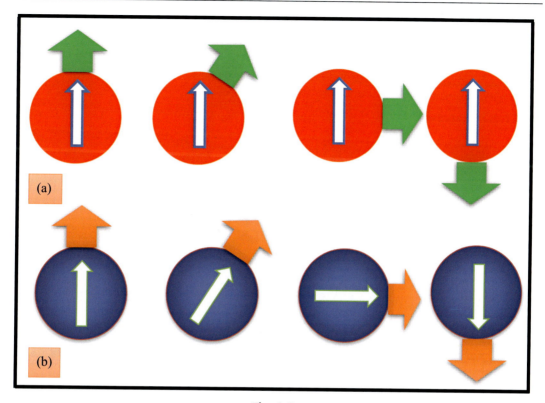

Fig. 3.2
(A) Visual representation of Neel relaxation (the particle is stationary but magnetic moment is rotating) and (B) Brownian relaxation (the magnetic moment is fixed but particle rotates).

3.7 Heat dissipation by MNPs

In MFH, the tumor is heated from "inside out." For better heating, MFH requires a higher concentration at the tumor site, which can only be obtained through directly injecting nanofluid in the tumor instead of an intravenous approach.

The heat released by MNPs under AMF with frequency f and strength H is demonstrated by the R. E. Rosensweig formulation [14]:

$$Q_{np} = \pi \mu_0 H^2 f \ddot{\chi} \quad (3.27)$$

where $\mu_0 = 4\pi \times 10^{-7}$ Tm/A represents the permeability of free space, $\ddot{\chi}$ is the loss component of the magnetic susceptibility χ given by the relation,

$$\ddot{\chi} = \left[\frac{\omega \tau}{1 + (\omega \tau)^2}\right] \chi_0 = \left[\frac{2\pi f \tau}{1 + (2\pi f \tau)^2}\right] \chi_0 \quad (3.28)$$

where χ_0 is the equilibrium susceptibility assumed to be chord susceptibility corresponding to the Langevin equation,

$$L(\xi) = \frac{M}{M_s} = \coth\left(\xi - \frac{1}{\xi}\right) \tag{3.29}$$

and can be expressed as

$$\chi_0 = \chi_i \frac{3}{\xi}\left[\coth\xi - \frac{1}{\xi}\right], \xi = \frac{\mu_0 M_d H V_M}{k_B T} \tag{3.30}$$

where χ_i is the initial susceptibility given by

$$\chi_i = \frac{\mu_0 M_d^2 \phi V_M}{3 k_B T} \tag{3.31}$$

here, M_d is the domain magnetization and $k = 1.38 \times 10^{-23}$ J/K is the Boltzmann constant. In Eq. (3.28), τ is the effective relaxation time given by

$$\frac{1}{\tau} = \frac{1}{\tau_N} + \frac{1}{\tau_B} \tag{3.32}$$

here, τ_N and τ_B are the Neel relaxation and Brownian relaxation time constants and are given by

$$\tau_N = \frac{\sqrt{\pi}}{2} \tau_0 \frac{e^{\Gamma}}{\sqrt{\Gamma}}, \tau_B = \frac{3\eta V_H}{k_B T} \tag{3.33}$$

with τ_0 being the average relaxation time in response to thermal equilibrium, η is the viscosity of nanofluid, T is the absolute temperature, and Γ is defined as

$$\Gamma = \frac{K V_M}{kT} \tag{3.34}$$

K is the magnetic crystalline anisotropy constant and, V_M is the volume of nanoparticles and is defined by

$$V_M = \frac{\pi}{6} D^3 \tag{3.35}$$

The hydrodynamic volume of MNPs is defined as

$$V_H = \frac{\pi}{6}(D + 2\delta)^3 \tag{3.36}$$

here, D represents the diameter of MNPs, and δ is the legend layer thickness, which is the thickness of a sorbed surfactant layer. The volume fraction of MNPs is defined by

$$\phi = \frac{M_s}{M_d} \tag{3.37}$$

Therefore, Eq. (3.27) becomes

$$P = \pi\mu_0\chi_0 H_0^2 f \left[\frac{\omega\tau}{1+(\omega\tau)^2}\right] = \pi\mu_0\chi_0 H_0^2 f \left[\frac{2\pi f \tau}{1+(2\pi f \tau)^2}\right] \quad (3.38)$$

The SLP is given by

$$\text{SLP} = \frac{P(f,H)}{\rho} = \frac{\pi\mu_0\ddot{\chi}H^2 f}{\rho} \quad (3.39)$$

where ρ is the density of MNPs. The power released by MNPs is computed as the specific absorption rate, which is the power generated by MNPs per unit mass, and is given by

$$P = \frac{1}{2}\omega\mu_0\chi_0 H^2 \frac{\omega\tau}{1+\omega^2\tau^2} \quad (3.40)$$

where H is the applied magnetic field, ω is the angular frequency, χ_0 is magnetic susceptibility, and $\omega = 2\pi f$. The magnetic moment **m** of a cluster of MNPs is defined as

$$\frac{\omega\tau}{1+\omega^2\tau^2} \quad (3.41)$$

and leads to global maximum SAR. If $\omega\tau = 1$, then it is known as critical frequency and for $\omega\tau \ll 1$ the power becomes

$$P = \frac{1}{2}\omega\mu_0\chi_0 H^2 \quad (3.42)$$

and for $\omega\tau \gg 1$, it becomes

$$P = \frac{\mu_0\chi_0 H^2}{2\tau} \quad (3.43)$$

and SAR does not depend on frequency.

3.8 Different heating sources used in magnetic fluid hyperthermia

The main heating tools used in hyperthermia include radio frequency, heating, microwave radiation, ultrasound, laser photocoagulation, hot water tubes, infrared radiation, and excitable thermal seeds. Each of these approaches carries limitations. The waves generated by these techniques have inaccurate focusing due to hotspots and their penetration power is also not good. These techniques generally heat tumors from the "outside-in" and produce more power losses. Here MFH presents the solution to all problems [10,15,16] because it heats tumor from the "inside out." Not only MNPs, but different heating sources can also be incorporated to heat the tumor depending on the size, type, and nature of the tumor. We list a few of them as follows.

3.8.1 Radio frequency heating

This method uses radio frequencies above 70,000 Hz for heating.

3.8.2 Microwave heating

It converts electromagnetic waves into thermal energy.

3.8.3 Ultrasound heating

This phenomenon is based on absorption. The mechanical energy is converted into heat.

3.8.4 Infrared radiation heating

Light and electromagnetic waves of any frequency heat surface through absorption of light.

3.8.5 Laser heating

Lasers of varying intensities and wavelengths are used to heat the target tissues.

References

[1] Gerber R. In: Asti G, editor. Magnetic separation applied magnetism. Dordrecht: Kluwer; 1994.
[2] Zborowski M. In: Zborowski M, editor. Physics of magnetic cell sorting scientific and clinical applications of magnetic carriers. New York: Plenum; 1997.
[3] Binns KJ, Trowbridge C, Lawrenson P. The analytical and numerical solution of electric and magnetic fields. Wiley; 1992.
[4] Carslaw HS, Jaeger JC. Conduction of heat in solids. 2nd ed. Oxford: Clarendon Press; 1959.
[5] Stratton JA. Electromagnetic theory. John Wiley & Sons; 2007.
[6] Bíró O. Edge element formulations of eddy current problems. Comput Methods Appl Mech Eng 1999;169:391–405.
[7] Carpenter C. Comparison of alternative formulations of 3-dimensional magnetic-field and eddy-current problems at power frequencies. In: Proceedings of the Institution of Electrical Engineers: IET; 1977. p. 1026–34.
[8] Nakata T, Takahashi N, Fujiwara K, Okada Y. Improvements of the T-omega method for 3-D eddy current analysis. IEEE Trans Magn 1988;24:94–7.
[9] Preston T, Reece A. Solution of 3-dimensional eddy current problems: the T-Ω method. IEEE Trans Magn 1982;18:486–91.
[10] Ng EYK, Kumar SD. Physical mechanism and modeling of heat generation and transfer in magnetic fluid hyperthermia through Néelian and Brownian relaxation: a review. Biomed Eng Online 2017;16:36.
[11] Kneller E. Theory of the magnetization curve of small crystals. In: Encyclopedia of physics, 18. Springer-Verlag; 1966. p. 2.
[12] Néel L. Théorie du traînage magnétique des substances massives dans le domaine de Rayleigh. J Phys Radium 1950;11:49–61.
[13] Brown Jr WF. Thermal fluctuations of a single-domain particle. Phys Rev 1963;130:1677.
[14] Rosensweig RE. Heating magnetic fluid with alternating magnetic field. J Magn Magn Mater 2002;252:370–4.

[15] Kumar CS, Mohammad F. Magnetic nanomaterials for hyperthermia-based therapy and controlled drug delivery. Adv Drug Deliv Rev 2011;63:789–808.
[16] Datta N, Krishnan S, Speiser D, Neufeld E, Kuster N, Bodis S, et al. Magnetic nanoparticle-induced hyperthermia with appropriate payloads: Paul Ehrlich's "magic (nano) bullet" for cancer theranostics? Cancer Treat Rev 2016;50:217–27.

CHAPTER 4

Mathematical models of physical processes involved in magnetic fluid hyperthermia

4.1 Modeling nanofluid flow in the injecting needle

The nanofluid flow in the injecting needle is governed by the laminar flow formulated by the Navier-Stokes equations coupled with continuity equation demonstrated as

$$\underbrace{\rho_{nf}\frac{\partial u}{\partial t} + \underbrace{\rho_{nf}(u \cdot \nabla)u = \nabla \cdot \left(-pI + \eta\left(\nabla u + (\nabla u)^T\right)\right)}_{\text{Stationary}}}_{\text{Time-dependent}} \quad (4.1)$$

$$\rho_{nf}(\nabla \cdot u) = 0$$

where u is the velocity, ρ_{nf} is the density, and η is the dynamic viscosity of the nanofluid.

4.2 Modeling nanofluid infusion in the tumor interstitium

In hyperthermia, the pressure-driven nanoflow from needle tip to the tumor tissue will be modeled by the steady-state Darcy's Law associated with continuity equation and is expressed as

$$\nabla \cdot (\rho_{nf} u) = 0$$
$$u = -\frac{K}{\mu}\nabla p \quad (4.2)$$

where ρ_{nf} is the density, K is tumor permeability, and μ is the dynamic viscosity of nanofluid. The ICs include pressure and velocity being zero in both tumor and normal tissue. This model under the effect of gravity will become

$$\nabla \cdot (\rho_{nf} u) = 0$$
$$u = -\frac{K}{\mu}(\nabla p + \rho_{nf} g \nabla h) \quad (4.3)$$

The constant g represents the gravity effect and h is an elevation. The pressure, $\rho_{nf} g \nabla h$ appeared due to the gravity and is added to the pressure ∇p.

4.3 Modeling nanofluid diffusion in the tumor interstitium

The diffusion of nanofluid in the tumor matrix can be modeled through the convection-diffusion equation:

$$\frac{\partial c_i}{\partial t} + \nabla \cdot (-D_i \nabla c_i) + \boldsymbol{u} \cdot \nabla c_i = R_i \quad (4.4)$$

The term $\boldsymbol{u} \nabla c_i$ represents the convection term and R_i is the reaction rate, which is zero here. The symbol, c_i, represents the molar concentration, of each species i. D_i is a diffusion coefficient that can be calculated by using the Stokes-Einstein equation:

$$D_i = \frac{k_B T}{6\pi \eta r_p} \quad (4.5)$$

where η is the dynamic viscosity of the nanofluid, k_B is the Boltzmann constant, T is the absolute temperature, and r_p is the radius of an MNP. When the nanofluid flows in the porous medium, the diffusion constant becomes

$$D^k = D_0 \frac{L}{F\tau} \quad (4.6)$$

$F > 1$ is the shape factor that accounts for hindrance in the pores, L is the factor responsible for the hydrodynamic and steric reduction of the diffusion coefficient in the pore, and $\tau(\varepsilon)$ is tortuosity due to increased diffusion path length.

4.4 Modeling transfer of heat in the body tissue

The heat transfer in the biological tissue can be calculated using Penne's bioheat transfer model (PBHTM) [1] expressed as

$$\rho_t c_t \frac{\partial T_t}{\partial t} = k_t \nabla^2 T_t + \omega_t \rho_b c_b (T_b - T_t) + Q_{met} \quad (4.7)$$

where T_t is tissue temperature (K), ρ_t is tissue density (kg/m^3), c_t is tissue-specific heat (J/kg/K), k_t is tissue-specific thermal conductivity (W/m/K), ρ_b is blood density (kg/m^3), c_b is blood specific heat capacity (J/kg/K), T_b is local arterial blood temperature equal to 37°C, ω_t, is local blood perfusion rate (kg/s/m^3), and Q_{met} is local metabolic heat generation rate (W/m^3). For the heat transfer in the tumor tissue, we will use model (4.7) with the addition of terms Q_{np} and is formulated as

$$\rho_c c_c \frac{\partial T_c}{\partial t} = k_c \nabla^2 T_c + \omega_c \rho_b c_b (T_b - T_c) + Q_{met} + Q_{np} \quad (4.8)$$

where Q_{np} is a constant heat source and comes from the model (3.38). If the heat source is variable depending on temperature and concentration, then the above equation becomes

$$\rho_c c_c \frac{\partial T_c}{\partial t} = k_c \nabla^2 T_c + \omega_c \rho_b c_b (T_b - T_c) + Q_{met} + Q_{np}(T, c_{np}) \qquad (4.9)$$

The blood perfusion rate ω_c (kg/s/m^3) in the above equations is taken as constant but if temperature-dependent blood perfusion is considered then the PBHTM becomes

$$\rho_c c_c \frac{\partial T_c}{\partial t} = k_c \nabla^2 T_c + \omega_c(T) \rho_b c_b (T_b - T_c) + Q_{met} + Q_{np} \qquad (4.10)$$

4.5 Modeling estimation of a fraction of tumor injury

The degree of tumor injury resulting from the tumor heating will be modeled by Arrhenius kinetic model [2], expressed as

$$F(x, y, z, \tau) = A_f \int_0^\tau e^{-\left[\frac{E_a}{R_u T_t(x,y,z,t)}\right]} dt = \ln C(0) - \ln C(\tau) \qquad (4.11)$$

where E_a is the activation energy, A_f is the frequency factor, R_u is the universal gas constant, $C(\tau)$ is the concentration of healthy cells remaining after heating of a duration τ, and $C(0)$ is the initial concentration of healthy cells. The fraction of undamaged tissue is expressed as

$$\theta_u = e^{-F(x, y, z, \tau)} \qquad (4.12)$$

And a fraction of necrosed tissue is predicted as

$$\theta_d = 1 - \theta_u \qquad (4.13)$$

These are the basic models; however, with time we will modify these models according to our simulation problems.

4.6 Physical properties of the nanofluid

The properties of the nanofluid will be calculated using the following theoretical models:

4.6.1 The volume fraction of the nanofluid

The volume fraction can be computed using the relation [3]:

$$\phi = \frac{\left(\frac{m_p}{\rho_p}\right)}{\left(\frac{m_p}{\rho_p} + \frac{m_{bf}}{\rho_{bf}}\right)} \times 100\% = \frac{V_p}{(V_p + V_{bf})} \times 100\% \qquad (4.14)$$

where m_{bf} and m_p are the molar masses of the base fluid and MNPs, respectively. ρ_{bf} and ρ_p are the densities of the base fluid and MNPs, respectively.

4.6.2 Effective density of the nanofluid

We can compute the effective density of nanofluid using the expression [4].

$$\rho_{nf} = \phi \rho_{np} + \rho_{bf}(1 - \phi) \tag{4.15}$$

where ρ_{bf} is the density of the base fluid, ρ_{np} is the density of the MNP, and ϕ is the volume fraction.

4.6.3 Nanofluid's specific heat capacity

We can compute the specific heat capacity of nanofluid for the known values of heat capacities of MNPs and base fluid c_p and c_{bf}, respectively [4],

$$c_{nf} = \frac{\phi \rho_{np} c_p + (1 - \phi) \rho_{bf} c_{bf}}{\rho_{np}} \tag{4.16}$$

where ρ_{np} is the density of the MNPs, ρ_{bf} is the density of the base fluid, ϕ is the volume fraction, and ρ_{bf} is the density of the base fluid.

4.6.4 Nanofluid's thermal conductivity

We will use the following equation [5] to compute the thermal conductivity of the nanofluid:

$$k_{nf} = k_{bf} \left[\frac{k_{np} + (n-1)k_{bf} - (n-1)\phi(k_{bf} - k_{np})}{k_{np} + (n-1)k_{bf} + \phi(k_{bf} - k_{np})} \right] \tag{4.17}$$

For 3D MNPs, we will take $n = 3$. k_{bf} is the thermal conductivity of the base fluid, k_{np} is the thermal conductivity of the MNPs, and ϕ is the volume fraction.

4.6.5 The viscosity of the nanofluid

We will compute the viscosity of the nanofluid using the following equation expression [6]:

$$\eta_{nf} = \frac{\eta_{bf}}{(1 - \phi)^{2.5}} \tag{4.18}$$

where η_{bf} is the viscosity of the base fluid, and ϕ is the volume fraction.

4.7 Flux of the nanofluid

If the volumetric flow rate of nanofluid is $\dot{V}$, then the nanofluid's flux at the tip of the injecting needle with cross-sectional area A_{needle} is calculated by the following expression [7]:

$$\text{Flux}_{nf} = \frac{\dot{V}\rho_{nf}}{A_{\text{needle}}} \qquad (4.19)$$

where ρ_{nf} is the nanofluid's density.

4.8 Nanofluid's mass concentration

The nanofluid's mass concentration of leaving the cavity can be calculated using the following relation [7]:

$$\gamma_{nf}(x, y) = \phi \times \rho_{nf} \qquad (4.20)$$

where ρ_{nf} is the density and ϕ is the volume fraction of the nanofluid.

4.9 Boundary conditions (BCs)

There are two basic types of boundary conditions.

4.9.1 Neumann boundary condition

Such conditions are expressed as applied force, flux, or current. The flux conditions specify how the external environment interacts with the model. These conditions address the component of a vector or tensor in a direction normal to the boundary, per unit area of the boundary. Examples of the flux conditions include:

- **Boundary load** that acts as a stress on the boundary.
- **Heat flux** that acts as heat per unit area.
- **The normal current density** that acts as electric current per unit area.

The general inward flux is formulated as

$$q = h(T_{\text{ext}} - T) \qquad (4.21)$$

where h is the heat transfer coefficient and T_{ext} is external temperature.

4.9.2 Dirichlet boundary condition

Such conditions are often represented by constraints. These constraints specify the results of interactions between the model and surroundings. Constraints specify one or more dependent variables at the boundary. Examples include

- **Prescribed displacement** at the boundary of the solid object.
- **Wall** that specifies slip, no-slip, sliding, leaking, or moving boundary.
- **The temperature** at the heated object boundary.
- **Electric potential** specify electrode in the AC/DC model.

The general temperature boundary condition is formulated as

$$T = T_0 \qquad (4.22)$$

where T_0 is the prescribed temperature at the boundary.

4.10 Initial conditions (ICs)

Initially, we will consider the temperature in all domains to be the normal temperature of the body

$$T_0 = 37°C = 310.15 \text{ K} \qquad (4.23)$$

Similarly, the ICs for pressure, velocity, concentration, and flux will be taken as zero.

References

[1] Pennes HH. Analysis of tissue and arterial blood temperatures in the resting human forearm. J Appl Physiol 1948;1:93–122.
[2] Huang H-C, Rege K, Heys JJ. Spatiotemporal temperature distribution and cancer cell death in response to extracellular hyperthermia induced by gold nanorods. ACS Nano 2010;4:2892–900.
[3] Sharifpur M, Tshimanga N, Meyer JP, Manca O. Experimental investigation and model development for thermal conductivity of α-Al_2O_3-glycerol nanofluids. Int Commun Heat Mass Transfer 2017;85:12–22.
[4] Buongiorno J. Convective transport in nanofluids. J Heat Transf 2006;128:240–50.
[5] Hamilton RL, Crosser O. Thermal conductivity of heterogeneous two-component systems. Ind Eng Chem Fundam 1962;1:187–91.
[6] Brinkman H. The viscosity of concentrated suspensions and solutions. J Chem Phys 1952;20:571.
[7] Eagle S, Wadsworth S, Wnorowski A. Modeling an injection profile of nanoparticles to optimize tumor treatment time with magnetic hyperthermia; 2015.

CHAPTER 5

Mathematical modeling and simulation of magnetic fluid hyperthermia of liver tumor

The liver is the largest organ in the body which exists internally under your right lung. It is mainly divided into left lobe and right lobe. The liver cells are called hepatocytes. It has also small cells in the form of line cells called bile ducts which are responsible for the transportation of bile from the liver to gallbladder [1]. The liver circulates the blood in the body. It removes chemical waste and toxins from the blood. The whole blood travels through the liver therefore liver is easily accessible to the cancer cells. The primary liver cancer that grows in other organs of the body can affect the liver severely. The major types of cancers include hepatic adenoma, hemangioma, benign tumors, lipoma, nodular hyperplasia, leiomyoma, cysts, and fibroma [2] (Fig. 5.1).

Liver cancer is a major health issue, particularly colorectal carcinoma with 27,000 new cases diagnosed in the United Kingdom and 157,000 cases in the United States diagnosed annually [3] and causes more than 17,000 deaths [4]. Surgery can be applied to a few cases due to tumor location in depth [5], and transplantation is inappropriate due to lack of availability of liver grafts [6]. The heat in hyperthermia can be produced using a laser, microwaves, ultrasound, or MNPs [7]. Magnetic fluid hyperthermia (MFH) provides a solution to the problem due to confined tumor heating for its killing [8]. This treatment technique is superior to conventionally used approaches because it can produce heat in deep-seated tumors with minimum collateral thermal damage [9]. Generally, magnetite Fe_3O_4 and maghemite γ-Fe_2O_3 MNPs are used in hyperthermia treatments due to their biocompatibility [10–12].

Historically, Pearce et al. [13] used FEM analysis to explore the energy density during MFH of the tumor using Fe_3O_4 MNPs. They used a needle approach for injecting nanofluid and concluded that effective heating for tumor damage can be achieved at the magnetic field strength 34kA/m at 160kHz frequency. Sawyer et al. [14] used FEM to treat the tumor with iron-cobalt MNPs. They focused on the Brownian relaxation mechanism with MNP agglomeration. They neglected the viscosity of the carrier liquids. Candeo and Dughiero [15] used FEM in MFH using iron oxide MNPs of different sizes for predicting the temperature distribution. They also predicted the behavior of SAR with particle concentration by varying MNP sizes. Javidi et al. [16] used Fe_3O_4 iron oxide MNPs to investigate the impact of different velocities and gel concentrations on MNPs during hyperthermia. They concluded that as the flow rate injection is increased, the mean temperature drops. Lv et al. [17] used γ-Fe_2O_3 MNPs in MFH of cancer to

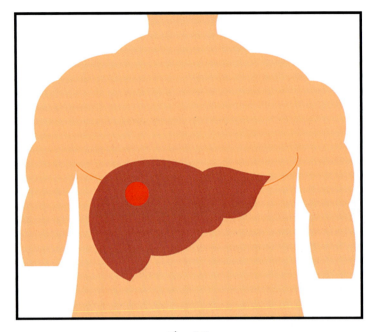

Fig. 5.1
Visual clue of human liver.

study the heat transfer in biological tissue coupled with external AMF. The studies [7,18] were performed using FePt MNPs in hyperthermia to treat cancer with promising results.

The MNPs utilized in the current study is made of a 3-nm coating of manganese ferrite ($MnFe_2O_4$) and a 9-nm core of cobalt ferrite ($CoFe_2O_4$), yielding a 15-nm core-shell MNPs: $CoFe_2O_4$@$MnFe_2O_4$. A typical representation of these MNPs is shown in Fig. 5.2. These MNPs

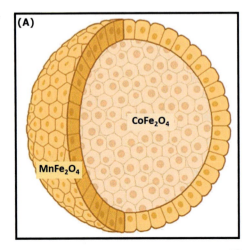
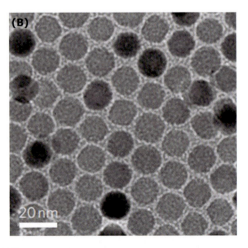

Fig. 5.2
Schematic diagram of core-shell nanoparticle with $MnFe_2O_4$ coating and $CoFe_2O_4$ core.

were synthesized by Lee et al. [19] through the modification of the growth method. The MNPs of size <100nm suspended in the base fluids like heavy water, propylene glycol, or ethylene glycol form the nanofluid. In the last decade, nanofluids have attracted the attention of scientific World community due to their enhanced thermal properties [20].

The density of $CoFe_2O_4$@$MnFe_2O_4$ MNPs is ρ_{np}=5300kg/m^3 and volume fraction ϕ=0.0013. If the base fluid used is saline, which is generally used in the medical infusion process, then according to AVCalc Limited Liability Company, USA, its density is $\rho_{basefluid}$=2170kg/m^3. With these values, Eq. (4.15) implies the density of nanofluid $\rho_{nanofluid}$=2174.069 kg/m^3. Substituting values of $\rho_{nanofluid}$=2174.069kg/m^3, $\dot{V}$=3μL/min, and A_{needle}=$\pi(0.000686m)^2$ in Eq. (4.19), we get $flux_{nanofluid}$=1.225kg/(m^2 s). The molar masses of $CoFe_2O_4$ and $MnFe_2O_4$ are M_c=234.6208 g/mol and M_s=230.6256 g/mol, respectively. The diameters of $CoFe_2O_4$ and $MnFe_2O_4$ are, respectively, D_c=9nm and D_s=15nm. The volume of core and nanoparticles are V_c=382nm^3 and V_{np}=1767nm^3, respectively. Therefore, the volume of the shell is V_s=$V_{np}-V_c$=1385nm^3. The percentages of the core and shell volumes to the total volume of nanoparticles are V_c/V_{np}=22% and V_s/V_{np}=78%, respectively. The molar mass of core-shell nanoparticles is %$V_c \times M_c$+%$V_s \times M_s$=231.5g/mol≈0.2315kg/mol and the molar mass of saline is 76.45g/mol. Therefore, the molar mass of nanofluid is 307.94g/mol. Consequently, the $flux_{nanofluid}$=7.35×10^{-5} kg/s/m^2 ≈ 3.18 × 10^{-4} mol/s/m^2. The details of all calculations can be found in Supplementary material: Appendix A.

5.1 Mathematical modeling formulation of the problem

The mathematical models that will deal with all the hyperthermia process are narrated below.

5.1.1 Nanofluid injection in the tumor

The pressure-driven nanofluid flow from the needle tip to the tumor interstitium is modeled by steady-state Darcy's Law coupled with mass conservation principle and is expressed by Eq. (4.2). The IC includes both the pressure and velocity being zero at the start of the process in all domains. The BC include the zero pressure at the outer boundary of normal liver tissue

$$p = 0 \quad (5.1)$$

and the pressure gradient is equal to zero where the needle shaft contacts the tissue due to insulation.

$$\nabla p = 0 \quad (5.2)$$

Also from Eq. (4.2) we have

$$\nabla^2 p = 0 \quad (5.3)$$

where p is a function of x and y. Therefore, the above equation becomes

$$p_{xx} + p_{yy} = 0 \quad (5.4)$$

To solve the above equation using separation of variables, let

$$p(x, y) = F(x)G(y) \tag{5.5}$$

be the solution of Eq. (5.4) and it gives

$$\ddot{F}(x)G(y) + F(x)\ddot{G}(y) = 0 \tag{5.6}$$

Rearranging Eq. (5.6) and equating them with a constant k

$$\frac{\ddot{F}(x)}{F(x)} = -\frac{\ddot{F}(x)}{G(y)} = -k^2 \, (say) \tag{5.7}$$

Eq. (5.7) implies two equations

$$\ddot{F}(x) + k^2 F(x) = 0 \tag{5.8}$$

$$\ddot{G}(x) - k^2 G(x) = 0 \tag{5.9}$$

Eqs. (5.8), (5.9) constitutes the solutions

$$F(x) = A\cos(kx) + B\sin(kx) \tag{5.10}$$

$$G(y) = Ce^{-ky} + De^{ky} \tag{5.11}$$

Solution (5.5) becomes

$$p(x, y) = (A\cos(kx) + B\sin(kx))(Ce^{-ky} + De^{ky}) \tag{5.12}$$

5.1.2 Nanofluid diffusion in the tumor

After injecting the nanofluid into the tumor, the MNPs form the cavity near the needle tip and the MNPs start to diffuse within the tumor, which we modeled through the convection-diffusion Eq. (4.4) where the diffusion coefficient is defined by the Stokes-Einstein Eq. (4.5). Substituting the values of $k_B = 1.38 \times 10^{-23}$ J/K, viscosity of solution, $\eta = 1.23 \times 10^{-3}$ Pa s, $T = 310.15$ K, and $r_p = 7.5$ nm, we get diffusion coefficient of nanofluid as $D_i = 2.4816 \times 10^{-11}$ m^2/s. Initially, there was no concentration in all domains and the BC includes the mass concentration at the needle tip defined by Eq. (4.18). Using values of $\rho_{nanofluid} = 2174.069$ kg/m^3 and $\phi = 0.0013$, the mass concentration at which the nanofluid leaves the needle is calculated as $\gamma_{np}(x,y) = \phi \times \rho_{nanofluid} = 2.83$ kg/m$^3 \approx 9.178$ mol/m^3.

5.1.3 Heat dissipation by the MNPs

Heating in magnetic materials by high-frequency magnetic fields can be generated through (a) hysteresis loss, (b) eddy currents, (c) Brownian relaxation, and (d) Neel relaxation. For superparamagnetic MNPs (diameter < 100 nm), the major contribution for heat loss is via Neel

Table 5.1 The parameters used in heating phenomena.

Parameter	Description	Values	Units	Source
D	Diameter of NPs	15	nm	[19]
δ	Legend layer	1	nm	[16]
H_0	Magnetic field intensity	2.65	kA/m	[19]
f_0	The frequency of magnetic field	500	kHz	[19]
M_d	Domain magnetization	6.63×10^5	A/m	[19]
M_s	Saturation of magnetization	110	A/m	[19]
μ_0	The permeability of free space	$4\pi \times 10^{-7}$	N/A^2	[19]
k_B	Boltzmann constant	1.38×10^{-23}	J/K	[19]
k	Thermal conductivity	5.3×10^6	W/m/K	[19]
K	Magnetic anisotropy constant	1.5×10^4	J/m^3	[19]
η	Dynamic viscosity of nanofluid	1.22×10^{-3}	Pa·s	[19]
ρ	Density of NPs	5300	kg/m^3	[19]
ϕ	Volume fraction of NPs	0.0013	–	[19]

and Brownian relaxations [21]. The power dissipation of MNPs under the impact of applied AC magnetic field, $H=H_0 \cos(\omega t)$ with strength H_0 and angular frequency $\omega=2\pi f$ is given by the R.E. Rosensweig formulation demonstrated by Eq. (3.38) which is based on Eqs. (3.28)–(3.37). The heat dissipation by the MNPs from Eq. (3.38) for the constant heat source is calculated as $Q_{np}=4.8446 \times 10^5$ W/m^3. All the involved parameters are listed in Table 5.1.

5.1.4 Transfer of heat in the liver tumor tissue

The quantitative temperature distribution in the biological liver tissue can be calculated using PBHTM (4.8). The IC includes temperature being 37°C in all domains. The boundary condition includes thermal insulation between tissue and needle

$$-\boldsymbol{n} \cdot (-k\nabla T) = 0 \quad (5.13)$$

The external boundary of the liver is subjected to the convective flux boundary condition

$$-\boldsymbol{n} \cdot (-k\nabla T) = h(T_{ext} - T) \quad (5.14)$$

where $h=200$ W/K/m^2 is the heat transfer coefficient and $T_{ext}=37$°C. All the physical and physiological properties of the liver and bioheat model are listed in Table 5.2.

5.1.5 Estimation of the fraction of tissue necrosis

The destruction of tumor cells is modeled by Arrhenius kinetic model (4.13). The fraction of the tumor damage is predicted using this model. The parametric values contributing to this model are listed in Table 5.3.

Table 5.2 Parameters used in the bioheat model and properties of the liver.

Parameter	Description	Values	Units	Source
T_b	Arterial blood temperature	37	°C	[22]
C_b	Specific heat of blood	3500	J/kg/K	[22]
ω_b	Blood perfusion rate	0.0151	1/s	[22]
ρ_b	Density of blood	1050	kg/m^3	[22]
Q_{met}	Metabolic heat	10,713	W/m^3	[22]
C_p	Heat capacity	3500	J/kg/K	[22]
ρ	Density	5300	kg/m^3	[19]
k	Thermal conductivity	0.642	W/m/K	[22]

Table 5.3 Parameters used in the Arrhenius kinetic model.

Parameter	Symbol	Cancer cells	Units	Source
A	Frequency factor	1.8×10^{36}	1/s	[22]
E_a	Activation energy	2.38×10^5	J/mol	[22]
R_u	Universal gas constant	8.23	J/mol/K	[22]

5.1.6 Heat sources in terms of concentration and temperature

By substituting Eqs. (3.28), (3.30), (3.31) in Eq. (3.38), one gets the following equation

$$Q_{np}(T, \phi) = \pi\mu_0 H_0^2 f \left[\frac{\omega\tau}{1+(\omega\tau)^2} \right] \left(\frac{\mu_0 M_d^2 \phi V_M}{3k_B T} \right) \frac{3}{\left(\frac{\mu_0 M_d H V_M}{k_B T} \right)} \left[\coth\left(\frac{\mu_0 M_d H V_M}{k_B T} \right) - \frac{1}{\left(\frac{\mu_0 M_d H V_M}{k_B T} \right)} \right] \tag{5.15}$$

Simplifying the above equation we get

$$Q_{np}(T, \phi) = \pi\mu_0 H_0^2 f \left[\frac{\omega\tau}{1+(\omega\tau)^2} \right] \phi \left(\frac{M_d}{H} \right) \left[\coth\left(\frac{\mu_0 M_d H V_M}{k_B T} \right) - \frac{1}{\left(\frac{\mu_0 M_d H V_M}{k_B T} \right)} \right] \tag{5.16}$$

Substituting Eq. (4.20) in Eq. (5.16), we get

$$Q_{np}(T, \gamma_{np}) = \pi\mu_0 H_0^2 f \left[\frac{\omega\tau}{1+(\omega\tau)^2} \right] \left(\frac{\gamma_{np}}{\rho_{np}} \right) \left(\frac{M_d}{H} \right) \left[\coth\left(\frac{\mu_0 M_d H V_M}{k_B T} \right) - \frac{1}{\left(\frac{\mu_0 M_d H V_M}{k_B T} \right)} \right] \tag{5.17}$$

Eq. (5.17) is nonlinear, to linearized this equation, we proceed as follows. To simplify the above equation, let

$$\beta = \frac{\mu_0 M_d H V_M}{k_B}$$

Eq. (5.17) becomes

$$Q_{np}(T, \gamma_{np}) = \pi\mu_0 H_0^2 f \left[\frac{\omega\tau}{1+(\omega\tau)^2}\right]\left(\frac{\gamma_{np}}{\rho_{np}}\right)\left(\frac{M_d}{H}\right)\left[\coth\left(\frac{\beta}{T}\right) - \left(\frac{T}{\beta}\right)\right] \quad (5.18)$$

Using Taylor series, the linearization of the above function of two variables at point ($T=T_a$, $\gamma_{np}=\gamma_{npa}$) is expressed by

$$Q_{np}(T, \gamma_{np}) = [Q_{np}(T, \gamma_{np})]_{\substack{T=T_a \\ \gamma_{np}=\gamma_{npa}}} + \left[\frac{\partial Q_{np}}{\partial T}\right]_{\substack{T=T_a \\ \gamma_{np}=\gamma_{npa}}}(T-T_a)$$

$$+ \left[\frac{\partial Q_{np}}{\partial \gamma_{np}}\right]_{\substack{T=T_a \\ \gamma_{np}=\gamma_{npa}}}(\gamma_{np}-\gamma_{npa}) \quad (5.19)$$

Taking derivatives of function (5.18), substituting in Eq. (5.19) and after simplification, we get the linearized equation (5.20):

$$Q_{np}(T,\gamma_{np}) = \pi\mu_0 H_0^2 f \left[\frac{\omega\tau}{1+(\omega\tau)^2}\right]\left(\frac{1}{\rho_{np}}\right)\left(\frac{M_d}{H}\right)\begin{bmatrix}\gamma_{npa}\left\{\coth\left(\frac{\beta}{T_a}\right)-\left(\frac{T_a}{\beta}\right)\right\} \\ +\gamma_{npa}\left\{\beta\operatorname{csch}^2\left(\frac{\beta}{T_a^3}\right)-\left(\frac{1}{\beta}\right)\right\}(T-T_a) \\ +\left\{\coth\left(\frac{\beta}{T_a}\right)-\left(\frac{T_a}{\beta}\right)\right\}(\gamma_{np}-\gamma_{npa})\end{bmatrix}$$

(5.20)

Since SLP is given by

$$\text{SLP} = \frac{Q_{np}}{\rho_{np}\phi} \quad (5.21)$$

Substituting Eq. (4.20) in Eq. (5.21) we get

$$Q_{np} = \text{SLP}(\rho_{np}\phi) = \text{SLP}\left(\rho_{np}\left(\frac{\gamma_{np}}{\rho_{np}}\right)\right) \quad (5.22)$$

This implies the following relation for heat source dependent on mass concentration.

$$Q_{np}(\gamma_{np}) = \text{SLP}(\gamma_{np}) \quad (5.23)$$

5.2 Results

Now we proceed toward our results obtained through simulations. To implement the whole hyperthermia process, we used COMSOL Multiphysics software. Firstly, we constructed an artificial geometry of the liver burdened with the tumor of a 10-mm diameter. A needle of

15-gauge with outer diameter 1.829 mm, inner diameter 1.372 mm, and needle wall width 0.23 mm was produced with the needle tip located at the tumor center. The liver is constructed using eight bezier polygon segments of the quadratic type. The whole geometry is demonstrated in Fig. 5.3A and the needle with exact dimensions is shown in Fig. 5.3B.

The nanofluid is injected using the needle into the liver tumor following Darcy's law. Therefore, we select first the physics of the problem as Darcy's law with the stationary study. Under hydraulic pressure, the tissue adjacent to the needle drifts away and forms a cavity near the needle tip. The nanofluid starts to diffuse throughout the liver tissue. For this diffusion, we select the physics of the convection-diffusion equation added from the transport of diluted species. The study for this physics was selected as time-dependent for transient analysis. To analyze the transfer of heat transfer in the normal liver tissue, we selected the physics of the bioheat equation. In the liver tumor, we associate the heat source with the bioheat equation. For the study of bioheat transfer, the physics is chosen time-dependent. After adding all physics, we added material for all domains. For tumor and normal tissue, the material was selected as bioheat/liver and for the needle, wall material made up of steel is taken. Before solving all physics of the problem, the mesh is generated in extra finer mesh mode demonstrated in Fig. 5.4. The number of degrees of freedom was 11,562 with the solution time as 1 min 15 s.

The steady-state nanofluid flow from the needle tip to the tumor is simulated in Fig. 5.5A. The maximum pressure at the needle tip is around 5.3 MPa and pressure at the outer boundary of the

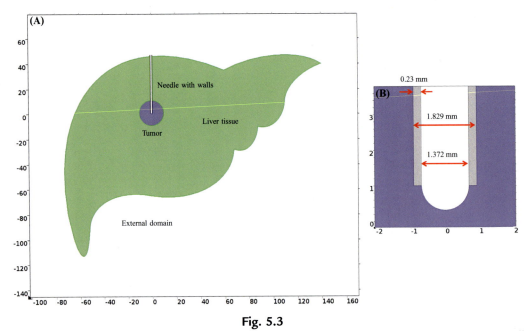

Fig. 5.3

Geometry of model: (A) Liver model with the tumor of size 10 mm and a 15-gauge injecting needle inserted at the center of the tumor and (B) injecting needle dimensions.

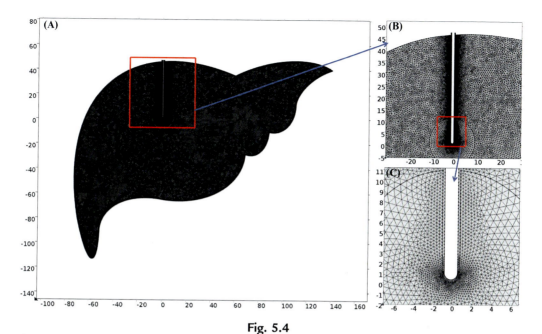

Fig. 5.4

Mesh generation: (A) the mesh has 70,815 triangular elements with a maximum element size of 1mm and a minimum element size of 0.00425mm. The numbers of boundary elements are 1341 and vortex elements are 24. Maximum element growth is 1.1 and minimum element quality is 0.5898, (B) the zoomed mesh of selective region in (A), and (C) zoomed mesh near needle tip for the selective region in (B).

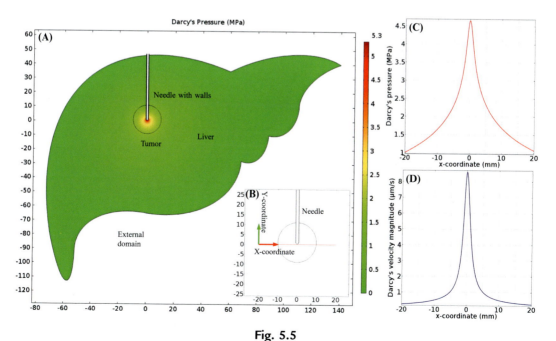

Fig. 5.5

Simulation of nanoflow from needle tip to the tumor: (A) 2D Darcy's pressure distribution, (B) visual clue of a line segment along x-coordinate, (C) Darcy's pressure distribution versus x-coordinate, (D) Darcy's velocity distribution versus x-coordinate.

liver is close to zero. To study the variation in velocity and pressure of nanofluid in liver tissue from the center to the radial outward direction, a line segment along the x-axis is drawn as demonstrated in Fig. 5.5B. Darcy's pressure distribution along this line segment is shown by a red curve as shown in Fig. 5.5C. The pressure distribution satisfies the Gaussian distribution curve and is symmetrical about the y-axis. The variation in pressure at the center of the tumor is maximum and is close to zero near the liver's outer boundary. We have also simulated the velocity profile along this line segment. The velocity profile also follows the Gaussian distribution curve as shown in Fig. 5.5D. The velocity at the center of the tumor is maximum and is close to zero near the liver's outer boundary. The maximum velocity at the needle tip is around 8.7 μm/s. The velocity curve behaves identical to the pressure curve but the velocity curve is steeper than the pressure curve.

The analytical solution (5.12) for pressure distribution is plotted in Fig. 5.6. The solution follows Gaussian distribution which agrees with the numerical solution of pressure distribution in Fig. 5.5C that also followed Gaussian distribution.

After injecting nanofluid into the tumor, the needle is removed and the nanofluid forms the cavity at the center of the tumor near the needle tip. Under injecting pressure, the nanofluid starts to diffuse in the radial outward direction. We have simulated the convection-diffusion Eq. (4.4) for formulating the time-dependent concentration of nanofluid. The concentration of MNPs after 24 h is shown in Fig. 5.7A. The maximum concentration is 9.18 mol/m^3 at the center of the tumor. The MNPs have been well distributed in the radial outward direction. In order to predict the concentration quantitatively, we select specific points x_i: $i=0.0, 0.5, 1.0, 1.5, 2.0$ mm in the tumor interstitium as shown in Fig. 5.7C. The concentration at time $t=9$h is

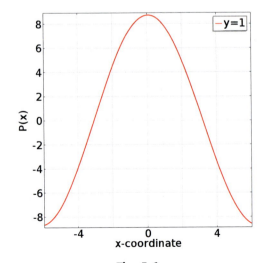

Fig. 5.6

Simulating analytical solution (5.12) for constants $A=B=2$, $C=D=1$, $k=1$, $y=1$.

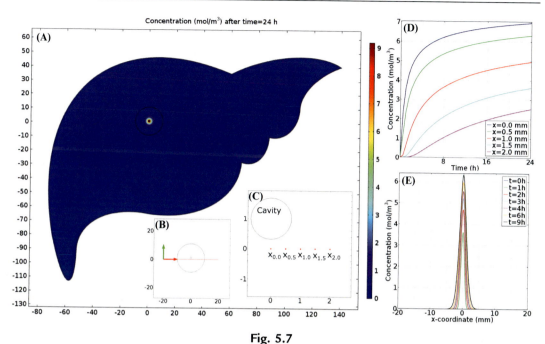

Fig. 5.7
Diffusion of nanofluid: (A) the concentration of nanofluid after $t=24$ h, (B) the visual clue of the line segment, (C) the visual clue of selected points, (D) the concentration versus time curves, and (E) the concentration versus x-coordinate curves.

higher than the concentration at time $t=0$ h. This result shows that concentration increases with increase in time and reaches maximum after 24 h. We also draw a line segment with the visual clue presented in Fig. 5.7B. The concentration against time plot at selected points is shown in Fig. 5.7D. This result shows that initially the concentration is zero and as time passes the concentration increases. After 24 h the concentration at $x=0$ mm of the tumor is 7 mol/m³ and at a distance $x=2$ mm from center of tumor, the concentration is 2.5 mol/m³. Thus as we move away from the center of the tumor, the concentration decreases. The concentration at the liver tissue's outer boundary becomes zero. Concentration along line segment with visual representation, is shown in Fig. 5.7B, follows a Gaussian distribution curve and is symmetrical about the y-axis. The concentration at the center of the tumor is maximum and minimum near the outer boundary of the tumor as demonstrated in Fig. 5.7E.

After diffusion of MNPs in the tumor that takes usually 24 h, the next step is to study heat transfer in the liver tissue. A magnetic field with the amplitude of 2.65 kA/m and a frequency of 500 kHz is applied to the distributed MNPs. Under Neel and Brownian relaxation, MNPs start to vibrate and produce heat. The heat dissipated by MNPs is calculated using Eq. (3.38) to be $Q_{np} = 4.8446 \times 10^5$ W/m³. This heat source is incorporated into the bioheat model (4.8) to study the transfer of heat in liver tumors. Before applying the magnetic field, the temperature in all domains was kept at the normal temperature (37°C) of the body. After applying the magnetic field, the temperature in the liver tissue is elevated. In the first 10–15min, the temperature is elevated to 45°C and after this, the same temperature is maintained till the end of heating time. The 2D temperature distribution in liver tissue is demonstrated in Fig. 5.8A. To investigate the temperature in the tumor quantitatively, we have selected points $x'_j : j = 0, 2, 4, 6, 8, 10$ mm as visualized in Fig. 5.8C. The temperature versus time plots at these points are simulated in Fig. 5.8D. After 60min, the temperature at distance $x' = 0$ mm is 45°C, and the temperature at a distance $x' = 10$ mm is 40.8°C. This result shows that the temperature decreases as we move outward from the center of the tumor. The maximum temperature is achieved at the tumor center and minimum at edges of liver tissue. The variation in the temperature along x-coordinate at selected times $t = 0, 0.5, 1, 1.5, 2, 2.5, 3, 3.5, 4, 10$ min is shown in Fig. 5.8E. The visual clue of the line segment is shown in Fig. 5.8B. The temperature curves follow Gaussian distribution. The temperature curves are symmetric about y-coordinate. The temperature at the tumor center is the maximum and is attenuated in a radial outward direction. As the time elapses from $t = 0$ min to $t = 10$ min, the temperature curves are shifted to the higher temperature. After 60min, the maximum temperature is attained at the center of the tumor and these curves start to attenuate on moving from the center of the tumor toward the radial outward direction and become minimum at the outer boundary of the liver.

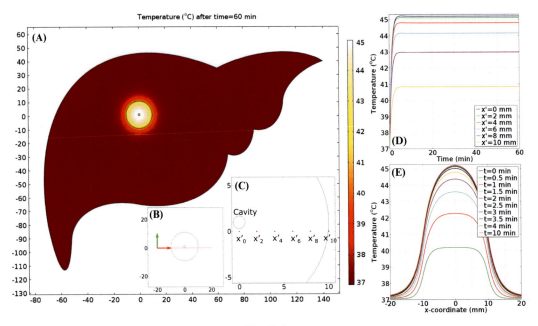

Fig. 5.8

Temperature distribution in liver tissue: (A) he temperature after $t=60$ min, (B) visual clue of the line segment in liver tissue, (C) visual clue of the selected point in the tumor region, (D) temperature versus time curves, and (E) temperature versus x-coordinate curves.

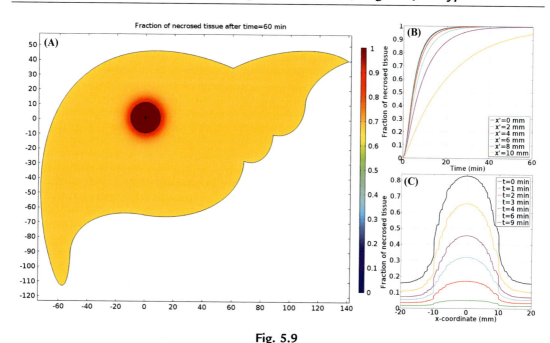

Fig. 5.9

The fraction of tumor necrosis: (A) 2D tumor damage after $t=60$ min, (B) the tumor damage versus time curves, and (C) the tumor damage versus x-coordinate curves.

To investigate the tumor damage quantitatively during hyperthermia, we have used Eq. (4.13). The 2D surface plot of the fraction of necrosed tissue predicted by this model is shown in Fig. 5.9A. For quantitative analysis of the tumor damage, we selected the five points with a visual clue shown in Fig. 5.8C. The point graph of the fraction of necrosed tissue versus time is shown in Fig. 5.9B. This result shows that after the application of the magnetic field, as time elapses, the tumor damage increases. The fraction of tumor damage is 1 at a distance $x'=0$ mm and this fraction is 0.92 at a distance $x'=10$ mm. Therefore, the tumor necrosis is maximum at the tumor center and it decreases as we move away from the center. The fraction of tumor damage versus x-coordinate along selected line segment and at selected times $t=0, 1, 2, 3, 4, 6, 10$ min is shown in Fig. 5.9C. The visual clue of selected points is shown in Fig. 5.8C. The fraction of tumor damage curves follows Gaussian distribution curves symmetric about y-coordinate. The tumor necrosis is maximum at the tumor center and minimum at the liver tissue's outer boundary. The nonsmoothness in tumor damage curves is due to the destruction of tumor cells.

For the validation of our simulations, we have compared our temperature versus time curves with that of Xuman Wang et al. [23]. This was an experimental study performed to investigate the heating effect of VX2 liver carcinoma of 10 mm radius in a New Zealand rabbit using Fe_3O_4 MNPs. The MNPs were injected into the tumor using a needle approach. After the diffusion, the magnetic field is applied to heat the MNPs. The temperature was measured at the center of the tumor using an optical fiber thermometer probe for 10 min (600s).

Validation of temperature predicted in the present study with this experimental study is demonstrated in Fig. 5.10A. These curves showed excellent agreement with the given experimental data. As an experimental data in a study by Wang et al. was available for only temperature versus time graph, therefore to validate the temperature versus x-coordinate curve in the present study, we have selected the study by Bagaria and Johnson [24] due to identical investigation, where they investigated the heating effect of MNPs in spherical tumor surrounded by healthy tissue in magnetic fluid hyperthermia. They predicted the temperature versus x-coordinate. The temperature versus x-coordinate in the present study is validated with the given analytical curve as shown in Fig. 5.10B. The agreement is excellent for given data and overall, our therapy works well. The experimental data of temperature versus radial distance in the study by Bagaria and Johnson was available for radial

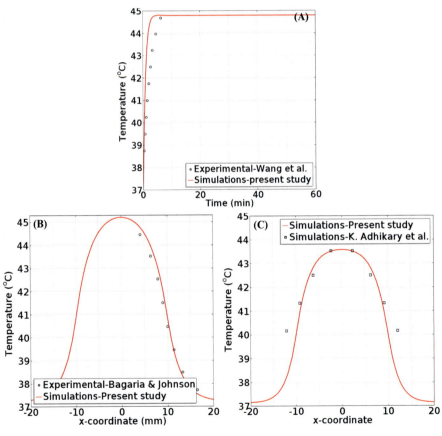

Fig. 5.10
Model validation: (A) validation of our simulation curve at a point selected in tumor near the center with available experimental data, (B) validation of our simulation curve along the x-coordinate of tissue with experimental data, and (C) validation of our simulated curve along the x-coordinate of tissue with K. Adhikary et al. simulation curve.

distance 0–20 mm and this demonstrates excellent agreement with our simulation for x-coordinate from 0 to 20 mm. Therefore, to validate the temperature versus x-coordinate curves from −20 to 20 mm, following the Gaussian distribution curve in our simulations, we have validated it with simulations by Adhikary et al. [20] as shown in Fig. 5.10C as well. Again, the agreement is excellent.

To show the superiority of $CoFe_2O_4@MnFe_2O_4$ used in our study over other MNPs we have selected a variety of core-shell MNPs and magnetite (Fe_3O_4) MNPs. Each type of MNPs is identified by its characteristics. We have selected all MNPs with the same size for comparison. The major parameters contributing to those MNPs to generate different heating effects are magnetic anisotropy and saturation magnetization as shown in Table 5.4. The temperature distribution curves generated by different heating effects of these MNPs versus time and x-coordinate are demonstrated in Fig. 5.11A and B, respectively. These results show that $CoFe_2O_4@MnFe_2O_4$ MNPs which we are considering in the present study for liver cancer therapy are superior to the $MnFe_2O_4@CoFe_2O_4$, $CoFe_2O_4@Fe_3O_4$, $Fe_3O_4@CoFe_2O_4$, and Fe_3O_4 MNPs.

Table 5.4 Properties of different MNPs [19].

MNPs	$CoFe_2O_4@MnFe_2O_4$	$MnFe_2O_4@CoFe_2O_4$	$CoFe_2O_4@Fe_3O_4$	$Fe_3O_4@CoFe_2O_4$	Fe_3O_4
Size of MNPs (nm)	15	15	15	15	15
M_s (emu/g)	110	108	105	104	101
K (J/m^3)	1.5×10^4	1.7×10^4	2×10^4	1.8×10^4	1.3×10^4

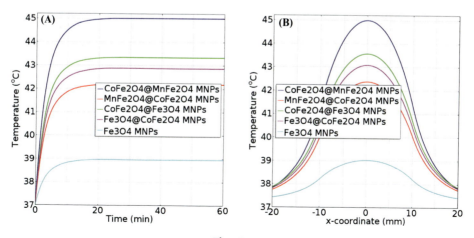

Fig. 5.11

Comparison of temperature distribution curves predicted by different MNPs: (A) temperature versus time curves and (B) temperature versus x-coordinate curves.

After this, the thermal analysis is performed taking into consideration constant and variable heat sources. The expression for power dependent on variable temperatures and concentrations is derived in Eqs. (5.17), (5.23), respectively. The temperature versus time curves for these two variable heat sources is simulated and compared with that of a constant heat source (4.8) as shown in Fig. 5.12. The temperature predicted by a constant heat source, temperature-dependent heat source, and the concentration-dependent heat source is 45°C, 45°C, and 47.2°C, respectively. This result shows that the concentration-dependent heat source produces a higher heating effect and consequently higher temperature as compared to the remaining two heat sources.

Eq. (5.18) represents the relation between the heat generated by MNPs as a function of concentration and temperature. We have plotted $Q_{np}(T,c_{npmax})$, $Q_{np}(T,c_{npavg})$, and $Q_{np}(T,c_{npmin})$ as shown in Fig. 5.13A–C, respectively. These results show that at maximum concentration, the generated heat is maximum.

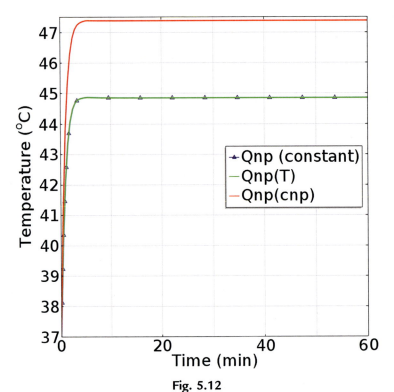

Fig. 5.12

Comparison of temperature predicted by three heat sources. Greenline represents the temperature predicted by the temperature-dependent heat source, the red line represents temperature predicted by the concentration-dependent heat source, and blue triangles represent temperature predicted by the constant heat source.

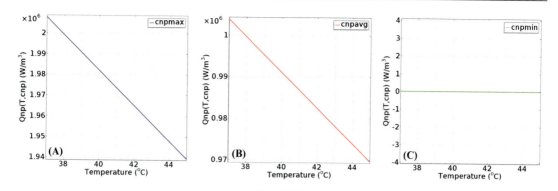

Fig. 5.13
Simulation of $Q_{np}(T, c_{np})$: (A) plot of $Q_{np}(T, c_{npmax})$ with $c_{npmax} = 9.178 \, \text{mol/m}^3$, (B) plot of $Q_{np}(T, c_{npavg})$ with $c_{npavg} = 4.59 \, \text{mol/m}^3$, and (C) plot of $Q_{np}(T, c_{npmin})$ with $c_{npmin} = 0 \, \text{mol/m}^3$.

The simulations of Eq. (5.21) are demonstrated in Fig. 5.14. Q_{np} is plotted against c_{np} at a fixed value of SLP of MNPs as shown in Fig. 5.14A which represents a linear relation. This result shows that as the concentration of MNPs is increased the generated heat also increased. The SLP is simulated against c_{np} at a fixed value of Q_{np} as shown in Fig. 5.14B. This result shows that SLP is inversely proportional to the concentration of nanofluid.

In the end, we have included the linearized plot of Eq. (5.20) as shown in Fig. 5.14. Since the linearized plot is a function of temperature and concentration, the simulated function is represented by both these variables. The temperature axis varies from 37°C to 45°C and concentration varies from 0 to 9.18 mol/m³ (Fig. 5.15).

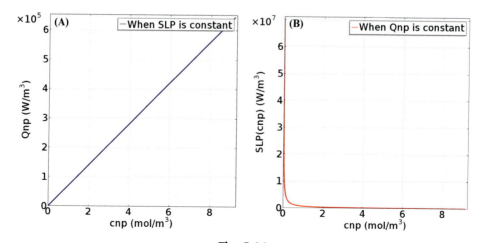

Fig. 5.14
Simulation of Eq. (5.21): (A) simulation of Q_{np} versus c_{np} and (B) simulation of SLP versus c_{np}.

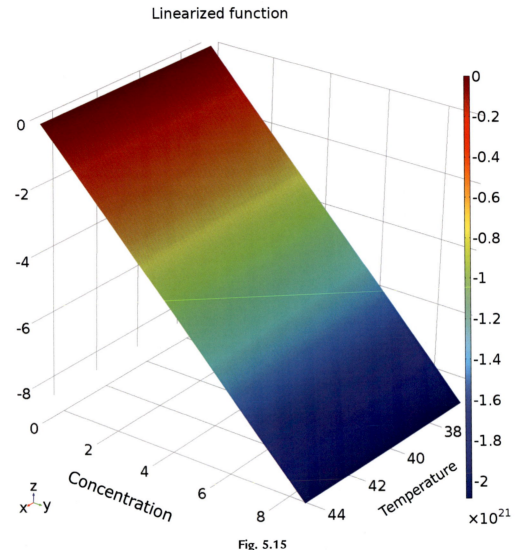

Fig. 5.15
Simulation of linearized equation (5.20): linearized function is dependent on T and ρ_{np}.

5.3 Conclusions

Core-shell $CoFe_2O_4$@$MnFe_2O_4$ MNPs are more effective for liver cancer treatment due to their superiority over the other MNPs. Both velocity and pressure of nanofluid during infusion in the tumor are maximum at the center of the tumor and decrease on moving away from the center. The concentration of nanofluid is maximum at the center of the tumor and minimum at the outer boundary of the tumor. Tumor temperature increases as the time of heating increases, and it is maximum at the center of the tumor and minimum at the outer boundary of the tumor. The fraction of tumor damage is maximum at the center of the tumor and minimum at the outer boundary of the tumor. Liver cancer is damaged with minimum collateral thermal damage. While comparing constant heat source with variable heat sources, the temperature versus time curves for the three heat sources reveals that the concentration-dependent heat sources produce more heat than the remaining heat sources. More heat is generated with increasing concentration for a given value of SLP and less SLP is generated with increasing concentration at a fixed value of heat. Our results agree well with preexisting literature. Thus, our therapy works well. We recommend using core-shell MNPs in hyperthermia of cancer in real-time treatments.

References

[1] Abou-Alfa GK, Jarnagin W, El Dika I, D'Angelica M, Lowery M, Brown K, et al. Liver and bile duct cancer. In: Abeloff's clinical oncology. Elsevier; 2020. p. 1314–1341.e11.

[2] Llovet JM, Fuster J, Bruix J. The Barcelona approach: diagnosis, staging, and treatment of hepatocellular carcinoma. Liver Transpl 2004;10:S115–20.

[3] Amin Z, Donald J, Masters A, Kant R, Steger A, Bown S, et al. Hepatic metastases: interstitial laser photocoagulation with real-time US monitoring and dynamic CT evaluation of treatment. Radiology 1993;187:339–47.

[4] Pestana C, Reitemeier RJ, Moertel CG, Judd ES, Dockerty MB. The natural history of carcinoma of the colon and rectum. Am J Surg 1964;108:826–9.

[5] Doci R, Gennari L, Bignami P, Montalto F, Morabito A, Bozzetti F. One hundred patients with hepatic metastases from colorectal cancer treated by resection: analysis of prognostic determinants. Br J Surg 1991;78:797–801.

[6] Bismuth H, Chiche L, Adam R, Castaing D, Diamond T, Dennison A. Liver resection versus transplantation for hepatocellular carcinoma in cirrhotic patients. Ann Surg 1993;218:145.

[7] Lin C-T, Liu K-C. Estimation for the heating effect of magnetic nanoparticles in perfused tissues. Int Commun Heat Mass Transfer 2009;36:241–4.

[8] Johannsen M, Gneveckow U, Eckelt L, Feussner A, Waldöfner N, Scholz R, et al. Clinical hyperthermia of prostate cancer using magnetic nanoparticles: presentation of a new interstitial technique. Int J Hyperthermia 2005;21:637–47.

[9] Gilchrist R, Medal R, Shorey WD, Hanselman RC, Parrott JC, Taylor CB. Selective inductive heating of lymph nodes. Ann Surg 1957;146:596.

[10] Hilger I, Hergt R, Kaiser WA. Towards breast cancer treatment by magnetic heating. J Magn Magn Mater 2005;293:314–9.

[11] Lazaro F, Abadia A, Romero M, Gutierrez L, Lazaro J, Morales M. Magnetic characterisation of rat muscle tissues after subcutaneous iron dextran injection. Biochim Biophys Acta (BBA)—Mol Basis Dis 2005;1740:434–45.

[12] Moroz P, Jones S, Gray B. Magnetically mediated hyperthermia: current status and future directions. Int J Hyperthermia 2002;18:267–84.

[13] Pearce J, Giustini A, Stigliano R, Hoopes PJ. Magnetic heating of nanoparticles: the importance of particle clustering to achieve therapeutic temperatures. J Nanotechnol Eng Med 2013;4, 011005.

[14] Sawyer CA, Habib AH, Miller K, Collier KN, Ondeck CL, McHenry ME. Modeling of temperature profile during magnetic thermotherapy for cancer treatment. J Appl Phys 2009;105:07B320.

[15] Candeo A, Dughiero F. Numerical FEM models for the planning of magnetic induction hyperthermia treatments with nanoparticles. IEEE Trans Magn 2009;45:1658–61.

[16] Javidi M, Heydari M, Karimi A, Haghpanahi M, Navidbakhsh M, Razmkon A. Evaluation of the effects of injection velocity and different gel concentrations on nanoparticles in hyperthermia therapy. J Biomed Phys Eng 2014;4:151.

[17] Lv Y-G, Deng Z-S, Liu J. 3-D numerical study on the induced heating effects of embedded micro/nanoparticles on human body subject to external medical electromagnetic field. IEEE Trans Nanobioscience 2005;4:284–94.

[18] Golneshan A, Lahonian M. The effect of magnetic nanoparticle dispersion on temperature distribution in a spherical tissue in magnetic fluid hyperthermia using the lattice Boltzmann method. Int J Hyperthermia 2011;27:266–74.

[19] Lee J-H, Jang J-T, Choi J-S, Moon SH, Noh S-H, Kim J-W, et al. Exchange-coupled magnetic nanoparticles for efficient heat induction. Nat Nanotechnol 2011;6:418.

[20] Adhikary K, Banerjee M. A thermofluid analysis of the magnetic nanoparticles enhanced heating effects in tissues embedded with large blood vessel during magnetic fluid hyperthermia. J Nanopart 2016;2016.

[21] Ng EYK, Kumar SD. Physical mechanism and modeling of heat generation and transfer in magnetic fluid hyperthermia through Néelian and Brownian relaxation: a review. Biomed Eng Online 2017;16:36.

[22] LeBrun A, Manuchehrabadi N, Attaluri A, Wang F, Ma R, Zhu L. MicroCT image-generated tumour geometry and SAR distribution for tumour temperature elevation simulations in magnetic nanoparticle hyperthermia. Int J Hyperthermia 2013;29:730–8.

[23] Wang X, Gu H, Yang Z. The heating effect of magnetic fluids in an alternating magnetic field. J Magn Magn Mater 2005;293:334–40.

[24] Bagaria H, Johnson D. Transient solution to the bioheat equation and optimization for magnetic fluid hyperthermia treatment. Int J Hyperthermia 2005;21:57–75.

CHAPTER 6

Modeling thermal therapy of poroelastic brain tumor using magnetic nanoparticles

The brain is an amazing three-pound organ of the human nervous system consisting of the cerebrum, cerebellum, and brain stem. The cerebrum is divided into two halves known as the left brain and the right brain. Each half of the brain has four lobes that include the temporal lobe, occipital lobe, frontal lobe, and parietal lobe. https://mayfieldclinic.com/pe-anatbrain.htm. It is a complex organ comprising 100 billion communicating nerves in trillions of signals. https://www.webmd.com/brain/picture-of-the-brain#1. People exposed to higher radiation in the head have more chances of developing brain tumors. People within an age limit of 65–69 years have a higher probability of getting brain tumors. A tumor initiating from the brain is known as benign tumors which is not very aggressive but is serious and life threatening. https://www.webmd.com/cancer/brain-cancer/brain-tumors-in-adults#1 (Fig. 6.1).

The brain tumor is a global health concern [1]. It is the growth of abnormal brain cells due to genetic and epigenetic events. It can be categorized into primary and secondary brain tumors. The primary tumor does not disintegrate and spread to other parts of the brain, but the secondary tumor spreads to the other organs of the body. A proliferating tumor eventually destroys brain tissue and slows down the normal functions of the brain. Gliomas are brain tumors that form 80% of all malignant tumors of the brain [2]. The World Health Organization [3] has classified gliomas into low-grade gliomas known as type I and type II brain tumors that look like healthy tissue and infiltrate slowly the normal brain ground tissue [4]. High-grade gliomas are known as type III and type IV brain tumors that look abnormal and proliferate rapidly and spread to large areas. This might produce a necrotic core, develop new vascularization to support growth, and convert the surrounding normal tissue to the tumor mass [5].

Glioblastoma multiform (GBM) and anaplastic astrocytoma are aggressive brain tumors where radiotherapy is the only option [6]. The chemotherapeutic approach in the treatment of tumor recurrence is also questionable [7]. Most of the chemotherapies are not able to penetrate through blood-brain barrier (BBB). It is also insufficient to reach such a concentration level with satisfactory brain therapy [8]. It also lacks to boost average patient survival [9]. Besides the BBB problem, chemotherapies possess low specificity toward cancer cells and cause aggregation in both cancerous and healthy tissues generating side effects [10]. High-grade

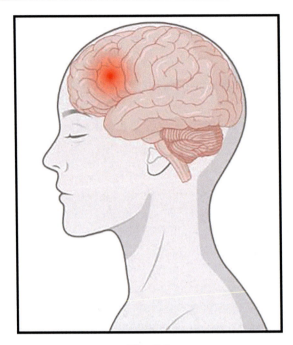

Fig. 6.1
Visual clue of human brain tumor.

conformal radiotherapy and 3D treatment planning also fail in the treatment of astrocytoma and alter the pattern of relapse [11,12] and when tumors are located where surgery is inaccessible then alternative options are needed [13]. Hyperthermia can induce selective heating in the tumors [14]. It is a therapeutic procedure that involves heat dissipation at the tumor site, where the temperature is elevated to 45°C, above normal body temperature of 37°C [15] and thus offers a solution to the problem.

Prominent research on brain tumor treatment from a mathematical modeling approach [16] includes the work by Pizzichelli et al. [17], who studied the infusion of MNPs in the brain tissue and developed an analytical model for time-dependent MNP concentration in the poroelastic tumor. Michele et al. [18] provided a quantitative framework for hyperthermia treatment designs. They took heterogeneous spherical tumors and derived analytical solutions for concentration during the infusion. Later, they computed the steady-state temperature distribution and justified the analytical results with numerical investigations. Basser [19] dealt with the analytical treatment of MNP infusion in brain tissue and modeled the swelling in a porous medium. Sobey et al. [20] simulated the nanofluid infusion tests in the poroelastic model to simulate the cerebrospinal fluid system. Su et al. [21] studied the effects of pore elasticity during the infusion process and comprehensively formulated the nanofluid distribution near the injected needle tip.

On the one hand, the literature shows that the limitation of the analytical approach is spherical symmetry. On the other hand, there are numerical studies that deal with thermotherapy, but their heating agents are not the MNPs, and they assumed the tissue to be in rigid form. Most of the studies also deal with the constant blood perfusion rate in the bioheat model. The lack of therapeutic approaches involving poroelastic tissue and heating tumor for tumor damage quantitatively motivated us to conduct this research. The objective here is to conduct and analyze the simulated results in an in silico study involving all the physical processes of hyperthermia treatment of poroelastic brain tumors using iron oxide MNPs as a heating source due to their good biocompatibility. We will incorporate temperature-dependent blood perfusion in Penne's bioheat model and will perform sensitivity analysis of selected parameters. The electromagnetic equations associated with the problem will also be simulated quantitatively.

6.1 Problem statement and strategy to handle the problem

A brain tumor of size 10mm (radius 5mm) is located in the brain tissue [22]. The objective is to damage this tumor with the minimum collateral damage to normal brain tissue. We are interested to model and simulate the whole thermal therapy of this tumor starting from nanofluid infusion in the tumor through injecting needle, diffusion in the tumor interstitium, and elevation of tumor temperature through heat generated by an external magnetic field to the prediction of tumor injury. How does the time-dependent blood perfusion behave instead of taking constant blood perfusion during this therapy? What is the impact of frequency and amplitude of applied magnetic field on the heating effect?

We will address this problem through our modeling strategy as shown in Fig. 6.2. In the current study, we are using the nanofluid consisting of iron oxide Fe_3O_4 MNPs with base fluid de-ionized water. The iron oxide MNPs being more biocompatible with unique magnetic properties [23] are attracting the scientific community due to their result-oriented applications in magnetic hyperthermia [24]. MNPs can have different shapes depending on the synthesis formulations. Fatima et al. [25] synthesized the iron oxide MNPs in the shape of cube, octahedron, and sphere using facile, safe, and convenient methods as shown in Fig. 6.3. The properties of nanofluid have been calculated as shown in Appendix B which will be later used in simulations.

The magnetic properties of Fe_3O_4 MNPs with different shapes were studied through magnetic hysteresis curves. All three types of Fe_3O_4 MNPs have zero magnetic hysteresis and as such superparamagnetic Fe_3O_4 MNPs possess such characteristics. The magnetic saturations were 87, 85, and 82 emu g^{-1} for spherical, cubic, and octahedral MNPs, respectively. The shape anisotropy plays a major role in changing the values of magnetic saturation [26]. Higher

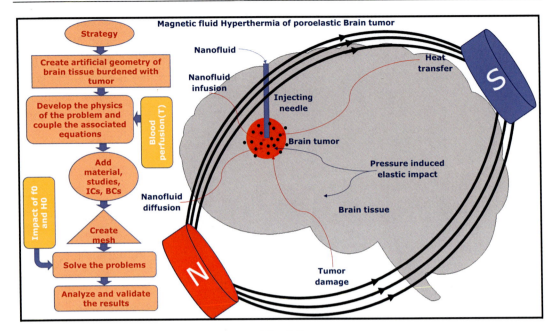

Fig. 6.2
Schematic representation of problem statement and solution strategy of the problem.

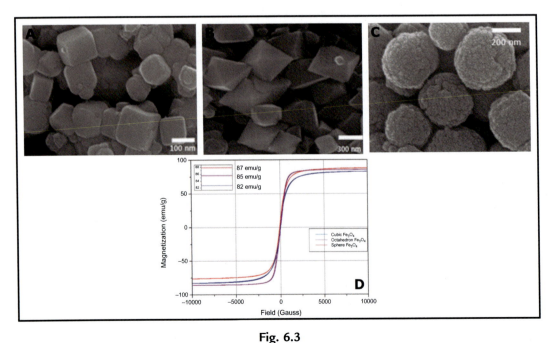

Fig. 6.3
Morphologies and magnetic properties of iron oxide MNPs: (A) cubic MNPs, (B) octahedron MNPs, (C) spherical MNPs, and (D) magnetization versus field profiles for MNPs with different shapes.

symmetry of Fe_3O_4 MNPs causes low magnetic saturation [25]. Therefore, spherical MNPs have higher magnetic saturation as compared to cubic and octahedral MNPs.

6.2 Deformation of poroelastic tumor

The pressure-driven injected nanofluid in the poroelastic brain tumor acts as stress and generates elastic deformation. The corresponding elastic strain and displacement are modeled through Biot's elastic theory [27–29]. The tissue is regarded as a combination of cells, interstitial fluid, and elastic fiber. It is considered anisotropic and compressible. Since we are considering a pore-elastic brain tissue, the most relevant numerical model is the pore-elastic model and is expressed as

$$\left.\begin{array}{r}-\nabla \cdot \boldsymbol{\tau} = \boldsymbol{F}_v \\ \boldsymbol{\tau} - \boldsymbol{\tau}_0 = \boldsymbol{C} : (\boldsymbol{\varepsilon} - \boldsymbol{\varepsilon}_0 - \boldsymbol{\varepsilon}_{\text{inel}}) - \alpha_B p_f \boldsymbol{I} \\ \boldsymbol{\varepsilon} = \frac{1}{2}\left[(\nabla \boldsymbol{u}) + (\nabla \boldsymbol{u})^T\right] \\ \nabla \cdot (\rho_{nf} \boldsymbol{u}) = 0 \\ \boldsymbol{u} = -\frac{K}{\mu}\nabla p\end{array}\right\} \quad (6.1)$$

The first equation of model (6.1) comes from Hooke's Law that formulates the stress and strain relationship. In the second equation of model (6.1), $\varepsilon_{el} = \varepsilon - \varepsilon_0 - \varepsilon_{\text{inel}}$ is the elastic strain which equals to total strain minus initial and inelastic strains, where τ_0 is initial stress, α_B is known as Biot-Willis's coefficient, and p_f is fluid pressure. The third equation of model (6.1) is the symmetric part of strain components and the last equation of model (6.1) is Darcy's law that will couple infusion of nanoflow with infusion-induced elastic deformation. In Darcy's law, ρ_{nf} is density, K is the permeability of the tumor, and μ is the dynamic viscosity of the nanofluid. The vector $\boldsymbol{u}$ (m/s) is the velocity of the nanofluid. The initial conditions (ICs) include velocity and pressure being zero in both normal and tumor brain tissues. The BCs include no flow condition for needle walls $-\boldsymbol{n}\cdot\rho_{nf}\boldsymbol{u}=0$, where $\boldsymbol{n}$ is a normal component of velocity and the mass flux leaving the needle tip is given by $-\boldsymbol{n}\cdot\rho_{nf}\boldsymbol{u}=N_0$, where $N_0=\text{flux}_{nf}$. The flux at the needle tip is $\text{flux}_{nf}=(\rho_{nf}\dot{V})/(A_{\text{needle}})$. Substituting the values, we get $\text{flux}_{\text{nanofluid}}=0.102\,\text{kg/(s m}^2)$. Nanofluid with a flow rate of 3 μL/min is injected at the center of the tumor. The total injection amount is 0.1 cc ferrofluid [21]. The other BCs include $p=0$ at the outer boundary of normal brain tissue and the pressure gradient is equal to zero where the needle shaft is in contact with the tissue due to insulation $\nabla p=0$. Moreover, during the infusion process, we assume the ratio of drained fluid volume to the specimen volume as $\alpha=V_d/V$, $0 \leq \alpha \leq 1$ [30]. The Young's modulus is $E=0.5\,\text{MPa}$, Poisson's ratio, $\upsilon=0.35$ [31], and porosity, $\varepsilon=0.2$ [32], therefore bulk modulus $K=E\upsilon/(1+\upsilon)(1-2\upsilon)$ and the shear modulus $G=E/2(1+K)$.

The permeability, $\kappa = 1.82 \times 10^{-15}$ m² [33], Biot-Willis coefficient, $\alpha_B = 1$ [28], and F_v represent inertial and body forces, which is zero in the current study.

6.3 Transport of the nanofluid in poroelastic tumor

The pressure-induced deformation causes the transport of the MNPs in the tumor. The transport of mobile nanofluid in the immobile tumor tissue matrix can be modeled by the solute transport model carrying convection, diffusion, dispersion, and sorption of the nanofluid within the poroelastic tissue. This model [34] is demonstrated as follows:

$$(\phi_p + \rho_b k_p)\frac{\partial c_i}{\partial t} + \left[c_i - \left(\frac{\rho_b}{1-\phi_p}\right)k_c\right]\frac{\partial \phi_p}{\partial t}$$

$$+ \nabla \cdot \left[-\left(\underbrace{D_i}_{\substack{\text{Diffusion}\\ \text{Coefficent}}} + \underbrace{D_d}_{\substack{\text{Dispersion}\\ \text{Coefficient}}}\right)\underbrace{\nabla c_i}_{\substack{\text{Concentration}\\ \text{Gradient}}}\right] + \underbrace{\boldsymbol{u} \cdot \nabla c_i}_{\text{Convection}}$$

$$= 0 \qquad (6.2)$$

where c_i is the molar concentration of each species i, ϕ_p is the volume fraction of the pores, ρ_b is the bulk density, ∇c_i is concentration gradient, $\boldsymbol{u} \cdot \nabla c_i$ represent convection, and D_i is a diffusion coefficient given by the Stokes-Einstein equation

$$D_i = \frac{k_B T}{6\pi \eta_{nf} r_p} \qquad (6.3)$$

where T is absolute temperature, k_B is Boltzmann constant, η_{nf} is the viscosity of nanofluid, and r_p is the radius of the nanoparticle. Substituting the values of $T = 310.15$ K and $\eta_{nf} = 1.72 \times 10^{-2}$ Pa s, and remaining values from Appendix B, we get the diffusion coefficient of nanofluid as $D_i = 1.76 \times 10^{-12}$ m²/s, D_d is the dispersion constant, and we assume shared dispersity in the current study. k_p and k_c are the Langmuir species constants and are defined as

$$k_p = \frac{k_L s_c}{(1 + k_L c_i)^2}, \quad k_c = \frac{k_L s_c c_i}{1 + k_L c_i} \qquad (6.4)$$

where s_c is maximum sorption and k_L is Langmuir constant. The IC is $c_i = 0$ and BCs are defined as no flux at the cavity boundary $-n \cdot N_i = 0$. The concentration leaving the cavity is $c_i = c_{0,j}$, where $c_{0,j}$ is the nanofluid's mass concentration. The nanofluid that leaves the cavity can be calculated using the relation $c_{0,j} = \phi \times \rho_{nf}$. Using values of $\rho_{nf} = 3006$ kg/m³ and $\phi = 0.6943$, the mass concentration at which the nanofluid leaves the needle is calculated as c_0,

$j = \phi \times \rho_{nf} = 2086.94 \text{ kg/m}^3 \approx 11,743.74 \text{ mol/m}^3$ from the cavity and the concentration at the outer boundary of the brain tissue is zero. We assume this concentration has a contribution from both sources; the concentration caused by an injected nanofluid and the small concentration caused by deformation in the brain tissue.

6.4 Heat produced by the MNPs in the poroelastic brain tissue

The heat dissipation by MNPs in alternating magnetic field is given by linear response theory (LRT) modeled by the Rosensweig formulation [35]

$$Q_{np} = \pi\mu_0 H_0^2 f \left[\frac{2\pi f \tau}{1 + (2\pi f \tau)^2}\right] \chi_0 \qquad (6.5)$$

All the formulas involved in the above model are discussed in Ref. [35] and the parameters involved are defined in Appendix B. Using these parameters, the power generated by MNPs is $Q_{np} = 4.73 \times 10^5 \text{ W/m}^3$. LRT is often used in the modeling of magnetic hyperthermia. It is not always valid in the case of magnetic hyperthermia, as often the employed magnetic field values are too high and the interaction between MNPs occurs. It is also only valid for the case $\mu_0 M_d H V_M \ll k_B T$. Diameter of NPs, $D = 15 \text{ nm}$, legend layer, $\delta = 1 \text{ nm}$, magnetic field intensity, $H_0 = 2.65 \text{ kA/m}$, frequency of magnetic field, $f_0 = 500 \text{ kHz}$, domain magnetization, $M_d = 6.36 \times 10^5 \text{ A/m}$, saturation of magnetization, $M_s = 110 \text{ G}$, permeability of free space, $\mu_0 = 4\pi \times 10^{-7}$ Tm/A, Boltzmann constant, $k_B = 1.38 \times 10^{-23} \text{ kg/m}^3$, thermal conductivity, $k = 5.3 \times 10^6 \text{ W/(mK)}$, and magnetic anisotropy constant, $K = 1.5 \times 10^4 \text{ J/m}^3$ [36].

The electromagnetic equations contributing to induction heating of brain tumor are

$$\left. \begin{array}{c} \sigma \dfrac{\partial A}{\partial t} + \nabla \times (\mu_0^{-1}\mu_r^{-1})B = \sigma v \times B + J_e, \; B = \nabla \times A \\ D = \varepsilon_0 \varepsilon_r E, \; B = \mu_0 \mu_r H \\ I_{\text{coil}} = \int J_e \cdot e_{\text{coil}}, \; J_e = \sigma \dfrac{V_{\text{coil}}}{d} e_{\text{coil}} \end{array} \right\} \qquad (6.6)$$

The first equation formulates Ampere's law subjected to magnetic vector potential. ε_0 and ε_r are absolute and relative permittivities and μ_0 and μ_r are absolute and relative permeabilities. I_{coil} is coil current, $n \times A = 0$ being magnetic insulation is BC at the outer boundary and IC is such that the initial value of magnetic vector potential $A = (0,0,0)$ Wb/m. We are supposing the dielectric properties to vary linearly with temperature in the healthy and cancerous tissues. The thermal conductivities and heat capacities are

$$k(T) = k(T_0)(1 + K_k \Delta T), C_p(T) = C_p(T_0)(1 + K_c \Delta T) \qquad (6.7)$$

where $K_k = 0.5\%$ °C^{-1} and $K_c = 0.33\%$ °C^{-1} and it may differ for blood due to high water content [37].

6.5 Heat transfer in poroelastic brain tissue

The temperature field in the brain tumor can be calculated using Penne's bioheat transfer equation [38]; together with heat generated by MNPs, the model becomes

$$[(\phi_p \rho_t c_t) + (1-\phi_p)\rho_{nf} c_t] \frac{\partial T}{\partial t} = [\phi_p k_t + (1-\phi_p) k_{nf}] \nabla^2 T + \omega_b(T) \rho_b c_b (T_b - T) + Q_{met} + Q_{np} \quad (6.8)$$

where $\omega_b(T)$ is the local blood perfusion rate, Q_m is the local metabolic heat generation rate, and Q_{np} is the heat dissipation by MNPs. The density of the white brain tissue is $\rho_t = 1041$ kg/m^3, thermal conductivity, $k_t = 0.48$ W/(mK), and specific heat capacity, $c_t = 3583$ J/(kgK). Arterial blood temperature, $T_b = 310.15$ K, specific heat of blood, $c_b = 3500$ J/(kgK), initial values of blood perfusion, $\omega_b = 0.003$ 1/s, density of blood, $\rho_b = 1000$ kg/m^3, and metabolic heat, $Q_{met} = 2708$ W/m^3 [39]. We will utilize this model to study heat transfer in brain tumors. The blood perfusion in the above equation is taken as temperature-dependent instead of constant. It is defined in Refs. [40, 41] for normal and tumor tissues and demonstrated in Eq. (6.9).

$$\omega_b(T) = \begin{cases} 0.45 + 3.55 e^{\left(-\frac{(T-45°)^2}{12}\right)}, & T \leq 42° \quad \text{Normal - tissue} \\ 0.833 - \left(\frac{(T-37°)^{4.8}}{5.438 \times 10^3}\right), & 37° \leq T \leq 42° \quad \text{Tumor - tissue} \end{cases} \quad (6.9)$$

The IC is $T_0 = 37$°C and BCs include thermal insulation $-\mathbf{n} \cdot (-k \nabla T) = 0$ and convective boundary condition defined as $-\mathbf{n} \cdot (-k \nabla T) = h(T_{ext} - T)$, where $h = 200$ W/(m^2 K) being the heat transfer coefficient and $T_{ext} = 37$°C.

6.6 The degree of tumor injury

The degree of destruction of tumor cells is predicted by the Arrhenius kinetic model [42] which is given by

$$\theta_d = 1 - e^{-\left(A \int_0^\tau e^{-\left[\frac{E_a}{R_u T_t(x,y,z,t)}\right]} dt\right)} \quad (6.10)$$

where $A = 1.8 \times 10^{36}$ 1/s, being the frequency factor, $E_a = 2.38 \times 10^5$ J/m the activation energy, and $R_u = 8.23$ J/(molK), universal gas constant [39]. In clinical practice, most studies report CEM43. The CEM43 dose model captures the heat-induced load feature on body tissue by predicting the equivalent thermal stress in minutes at 43°C. The thermal dose (CEM43) model accumulates temperatures above 39°C and calculates dose equivalent minutes at 43°C as

$$\text{CEM43}(t) = \int_{t_i}^{t_f} R^{(43-T(t))} dt \qquad (6.11)$$

where t_i and t_f are the initial and final heating times, respectively, $T(t)$ is tissue temperature, and R is constant equivalent to 0.5 for $T(t)>43°C$, 0.25 for $49°C<T(t)<43°C$, and 0 for $T(t)<43°C$. The tissues under heat exposer have damage thresholds: CEM43=15min for skin, fat, muscle, and bone tissues, CEM43=2min for the blood-brain barrier and brain tissues [43].

6.7 Implementation in COMSOL multiphysics

The geometry of the model is shown in Fig. 6.4. The tumor is assumed to be in the brain' white matter because the white matter is approximately one-third stiffer than gray matter and it has demonstrated large regional variations. It is more viscous than gray matter and showed longer

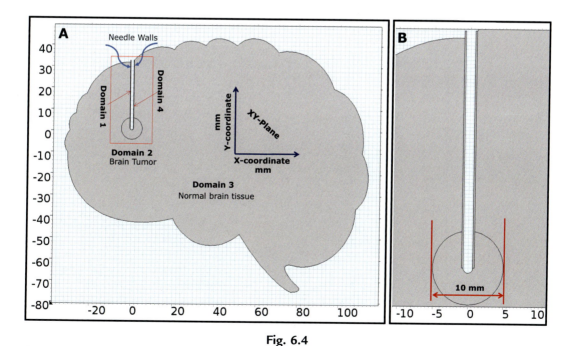

Fig. 6.4
The geometry of the problem: (A) 2D geometry of brain tumor with surrounding normal white brain tissue and injected needle with the tip at the center of brain tumor. (B) The needle has following dimensions: outer diameter 1.83 mm, inner diameter 1.732 mm, and needle wall with width 0.229 mm.

relaxation times. The rheological differences between gray and white matter have direct implications on diagnosing mechanical phenomena during neurodevelopment [44].

The material for needle domains 1 and 4 was added as steel AISI 4340 and for brain tissue, domains 2 and 3 as bioheat/muscle. The ICs and BCs for the physics of poroelasticity, convection-diffusion equation, and bioheat transfer model are added as mentioned in Sections 2.2, 2.3, and 2.5, respectively.

A mesh was generated in extra-fine mesh mode and convergence plots guarantee the convergence of the solution. The generated mesh is demonstrated in Fig. 6.5.

6.8 Results and discussions

In this study, we present a computational study of the thermal therapy of the brain tumor using iron oxide Fe_3O_4 MNPs. The whole hyperthermia procedure for a brain tumor has been simulated using COMSOL Multiphysics software for quantitative analysis. As the first step of the systematic study of a highly complicated process some assumptions are introduced: (i) the poroelastic tumor matrix is taken as isotropic, (ii) under equilibrium conditions, stress and

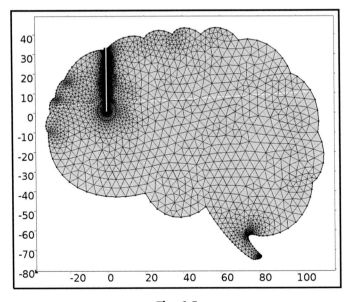

Fig. 6.5
Mesh of the model: mesh is generated in finer mesh mode with triangular elements. The complete mesh consists of 5928 domain elements and 631 boundary elements. The minimum element size was 0.0195 mm and the maximum element size was 5.73 mm.

strain relationships are irreversible, (iii) for small stresses, stress-strain relationships are linear, (iv) under stress, a small strain is produced, and (v) the nanofluid contained in pores is incompressible.

The infusion model is solved for pressure and velocity profiles. The 2D surface plot of pressure distribution is demonstrated in Fig. 6.6A. The pressure achieved at the needle tip is 0.61 MPa. The pressure of nanofluid at the needle tip is maximum but it is minimum at the outer tumor boundary. To investigate the pressure variation along the radius, a line segment is drawn with the visual clue shown in the lower left corner of Fig. 6.6A. The line graphs of pressure and velocity profiles of a nanofluid along the line are demonstrated in Fig. 6.6B and C respectively. Both the graphs are symmetric about y-axes with bell-shaped peaks. The maximum velocity achieved at the needle tip is 20μm/s. Although the behavior of pressure and velocity is identical the velocity curve is steeper than the pressure curve. Since the circular tumor is symmetric concerning an axial needle with a needle tip at the center, we get the symmetric curves of both velocity and pressure of nanofluid.

The elastic impact of nanofluid pressure on brain tissue is simulated in Fig. 6.7A. The deformation displacement is simulated. The deformation displacement is shifted throughout the brain tissue, especially nanofluid has the tendency to move in the backward direction from needle tip to the region adjacent to the tissue-needle interface and causes backflow. The surface

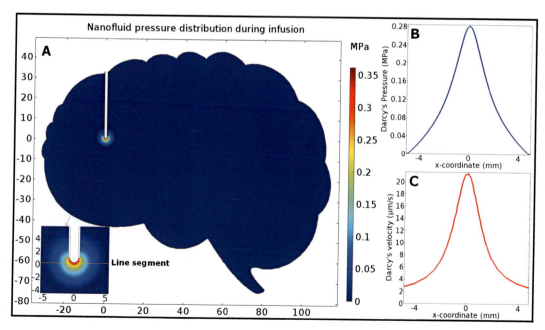

Fig. 6.6

Simulation of infusion of nanofluid in the tumor: (A) surface plot of the pressure distribution of the nanofluid, (B) Darcy's pressure versus x-coordinate, and (C) Darcy's velocity versus x-coordinate.

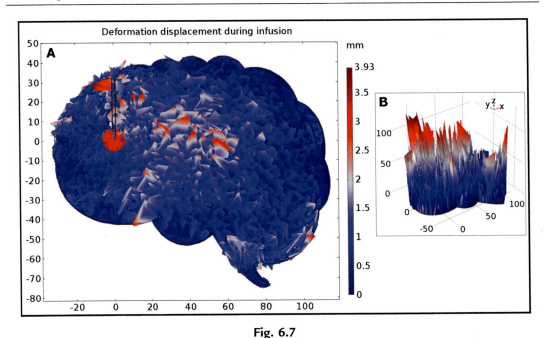

Fig. 6.7
Simulation of poroelasticity: (A) deformation displacement distribution in the brain tissue. (B) Surface with height plot of deformation displacement.

with the height plot of deformation displacement is demonstrated in Fig. 6.7B. The fluctuation in the plot shows the back and forth motion of displaced brain tissue.

During infusion, the poroelastic model (6.1) is solved for the stress of the nanofluid. The 2D stress distribution is shown in Fig. 6.8A. The maximum stress 84 MPa is achieved at the tumor center and is minimum near the out boundary of the tumor. The stress is maximum at the center and decreases in the radial outward direction. The stress is minimum at the outer boundary of the brain tissue. The corresponding strain caused by this stress is simulated in Fig. 6.8B. The graph of volumetric strain demonstrates fluctuating behavior due to the back and forth motion of the tissue.

After infusion, the injecting needle is removed and the deformation induced in the brain tissue causes the nanofluid to diffuse in the brain tissue. The diffusion of the nanofluid in the tumor is modeled through the solute transport model (6.2) and is simulated for concentration. To be more realistic, we have incorporated convection, diffusion dispersion, and sorption of the nanofluid in the transport model instead of simply dealing with the diffusion equation. The 2D concentration after time $t = 24$h is simulated in Fig. 6.9A. The concentration is maximum near the cavity and minimum at the tumor boundary. To investigate the quantitative behavior

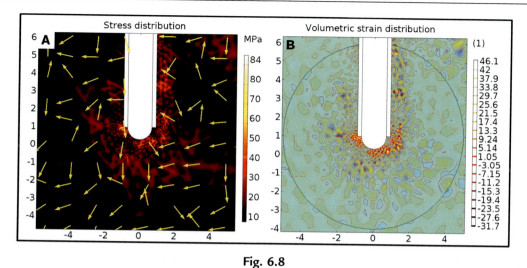

Fig. 6.8
Simulation of the solution of the poroelastic model for stress and strain: (A) 2D stress distribution. (B) Volumetric strain versus x-coordinate.

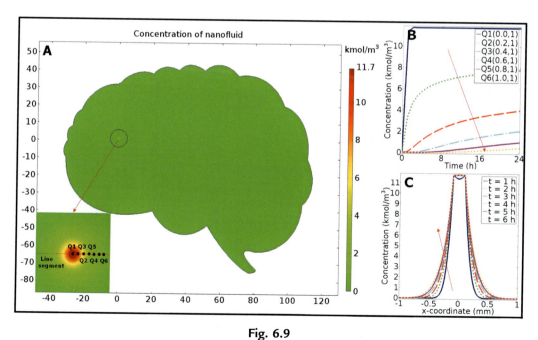

Fig. 6.9
Simulation of nanofluid concentration: (A) 2D concentration of nanofluid, (B) concentration against time profile, and (C) concentration against x-coordinate profiles.

of concentration inside the brain tissue we have selected five points $Q_i(x_i,y_i)=(0.0,1)$, $(0.2,1)$, $(0.4,1)$, $(0.6,1)$, $(0.8,1)$, $(1.0,1)$ mm with the visual clue of these points demonstrated in lower left corner of Fig. 6.9A. The point graph of the concentration against time at these points is shown in Fig. 6.9B. Initially, the concentration of nanoflow was concentrated to the cavity only but the back and forth motion of tissue due to the deformation effect, which was initiated due to injected pressure, causes the nanofluid to diffuse throughout the brain tissue. After time $t=24$ h, nanofluid is distributed inside the brain tissue and becomes broader and flatter. Moreover, the concentration at point $(0.0,1)$ is higher than at points $(0.2,1)$, $(0.4,1)$, $(0.6,1)$, $(0.8,1)$, $(1.0,1)$ mm. This shows that the concentration at the tumor center is higher than that at the outer boundary of the brain tissue. The graph of concentration along the line segment is demonstrated in Fig. 6.9B where the visual clue of the line segment is shown in the lower left corner of Fig. 6.9A. The concentration of the nanofluid is maximum near the cavity and minimum at the outer boundary of brain tissue. The concentration at the selected times $t=1, 2, 3, 4, 5, 6$h in increasing order shifts the concentration versus x-coordinate curves to more steep curves and with higher peak values. This result shows that at any point in the brain tissue, the distribution of concentration increases as the time elapses and it becomes maximum after 24 h. Moreover, the concentration profiles are symmetrical curves about $x=0$ line. After the needle is pulled out, we assumed the formation of the cavity of nanofluid at the tumor center. This nanofluid later distributes throughout the tumor region via injected pressure and stress forces. In the case of solid tumors, the injection of nanofluid may develop microcrakes in the tumor analog to the hydraulic fracture model [45]. But in the case of elastic tissue, there is the probability of leakage of nanofluid from the tumor, and this problem is termed as backflow problem [46]. To control that flow nanofluid should be injected at lower flow rates typically of 3 μL/min.

The bioheat model is solved for temperature estimation in the brain tissue. The temperature in the brain tissue after $t=60$ min is shown in Fig. 6.10A. The temperature is raised to 42°C inside the tumor from 37°C of normal body temperature. In order to investigate the temperature behavior quantitatively inside the brain tissue, five points $P_i(x_i,y_i)=(0,1), (1,1), (2,1), (3,1), (4,1), (5,1)$ are selected that are visualized at the lower left corner of Fig. 6.10A. The temperature versus time curves at these points are simulated in Fig. 6.10B. After the application of AMF, the temperature is elevated to 42°C within the first 10min. After this, the temperature becomes stable till the end of the heating time. The temperature at the point $(0,1)$ is 42°C and is less than 42°C at the remaining points. This result shows that the temperature at the center of the tumor is higher than the temperature at locations away from the center. The variation in temperature versus x-coordinate is simulated in Fig. 6.10C where the visual clue of the line segment is visualized at the left lower corner of Fig. 6.10A. The temperature curves at the selected times $t=0, 1, 2, 3, 4, 10$min follow

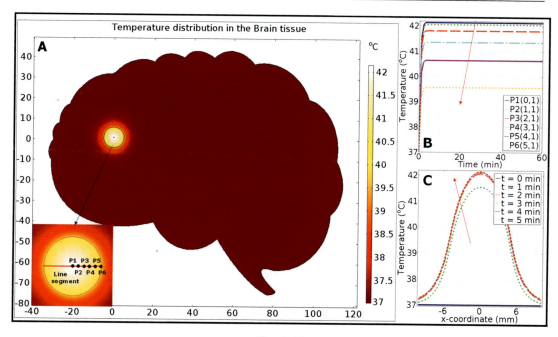

Fig. 6.10

Temperature distribution in the brain tumor: (A) temperature after time $t = 60$ min, (B) temperature versus time profile at selected points, and (C) temperature versus x-coordinate at selected times.

symmetric curves and these curves shift to higher temperatures with increasing time. This result shows that the temperature increases with time.

Now we will simulate the temperature-dependent blood perfusion model (6.9) coupled with the bioheat model. The simulation of temperature-dependent blood perfusion in healthy tissue is demonstrated in Fig. 6.11A. As the temperature increases, the blood perfusion in healthy tissue also increases. The blood perfusion shows periodic behavior. The peaks of the maximum values are obtained at the temperatures $45°C$ and $53°C$. The simulation of blood perfusion in tumor tissue is demonstrated in Fig. 6.11B. In tumor tissue, blood perfusion behaves opposite to the behavior in healthy tissue. Here the blood perfusion decreases with increasing temperature. Lower spikes are obtained at $42°C$, $47°C$, and $52°C$.

The degree of tumor injury is simulated in Fig. 6.12A. The tumor injury is maximum at the tumor center and minimum at the edges of the tumor. The fraction of tumor injury versus time at the selected points is computed in Fig. 6.12B. The selected points were the same as taken in temperature simulations. The tumor injury is maximum at the point (0,1) and minimum at point

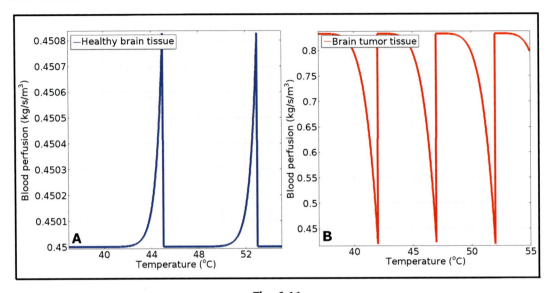

Fig. 6.11

Simulation of temperature-dependent blood perfusion: (A) blood perfusion in healthy tissue and (B) blood perfusion in tumor tissue.

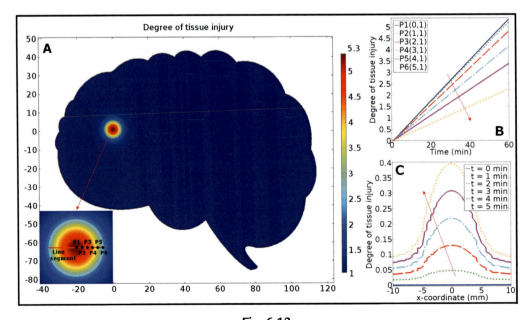

Fig. 6.12

Estimation of tumor destruction: (A) degree of tumor injury after $t=60$ min, (B) degree of tumor injury versus time, and (C) degree of tissue injury versus x-coordinate.

(5,1). Thus, more tumor is damaged at the center as compared to that at the outer boundary. The fraction of tumor injury versus x-coordinate at times $t = 0, 1, 2, 3, 4, 5$ min is simulated in Fig. 6.12C where the selected line segment is visualized at the lower left corner of Fig. 6.12C. With time tumor damage curves shift to the higher fraction which implies maximum tumor damage at the maximum time, $t = 60$ min.

For validation of our simulations, we have compared our temperature versus time curve with that of Lin and Liu's work [22]. In this study, the FePt MNPs were used to predict the temperature distribution. They took the size of the tumor as 10 mm. They used an analytical approach and a hybrid numerical scheme to solve the bioheat equation to investigate the heating effect in a bilayered spherical tissue and compared it with the analytical solution. In this work, a spherical tumor was considered surrounded by normal tissue. The validation of temperature versus time curves is shown in Fig. 6.13. In the current study, we are considering the tumor of the same size. We are also using MNPs as a heat sources. The tumor is also surrounded by healthy tissue. For comparison, we have to compromise over some parameters, however, we were successful to compare our results with existing literature. The availability of better experimental data can compensate for this compromise.

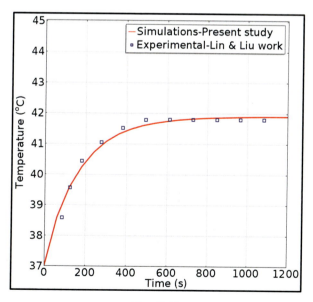

Fig. 6.13

Model validation: validation of temperature versus time profile. *Sold line* is simulation curve in the present study generated at $r = 5$ mm, $f_0 = 500$ kHz, and $H_0 = 37.4$ kAm^{-1}. The *squared dotted curve* is an analytical solution by Lin and Liu.

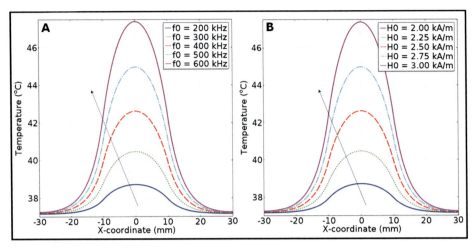

Fig. 6.14

Sensitivity of parameters: (A) impact of different frequencies on temperature distribution at constant amplitude $H_0 = 2.75\,\text{kA}\,\text{m}^{-1}$ and (B) impact of different amplitudes on temperature distribution at constant frequency $f_0 = 500\,\text{kHz}$.

There are many parameters involved in this study. So given their sensitivity, we are considering only the impact of amplitude and frequency of AMF on the heating effect. Among heating parameters, these two parameters mainly influenced the temperature distribution. This is also evident from the formula (6.5), where frequency f_0 and amplitude H_0 are directly proportional to the heat, Q_{np}. The impact of variation of frequencies f_0: 200–600 kHz with step size 100 kHz at constant amplitude is demonstrated in Fig. 6.14A. The result shows that as the frequency of the AMF is increased, the peak value of the temperature profile also shifts to a higher temperature. The impact of variation of amplitudes H_0: 2:00–3:00 kA/m with step size 0.25 kA/m at constant frequency f_0: 200 kHz is demonstrated in Fig. 6.14B. The result shows that as the amplitude of the applied magnetic field is increased, the peak value of the temperature profile also shifts to a higher temperature. Thus increment in the amplitude of frequency of the AMF will result in enhancing the temperature.

In order to simulate electromagnetic equations generating AMF to heat the tumor tissue, we have constructed a current-carrying coil surrounded by air domain as shown in Fig. 6.15A. The corresponding simulation of magnetic flux density is shown in Fig. 6.15B. The magnetic lines of force are distributed uniformly throughout the effective region for brain tissue.

Lastly, the induction heating of brain tumors is shown in Fig. 6.16. The current-carrying coil generates a magnetic field following Ampere's law. The magnetic line of force crosses the brain tissue burdened with MNPs and this heats the tumor due to Neel and Brownian relaxation effects.

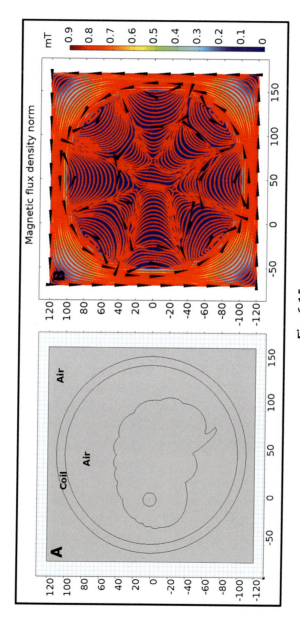

Fig. 6.15

(A) Geometry of the brain tissue enclosed by a coil with air domain and (B) magnetic flux density distribution.

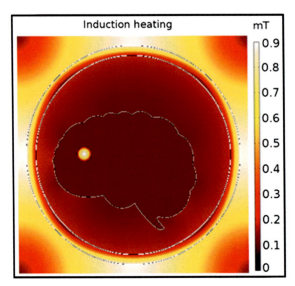

Fig. 6.16
Induction heating of brain tumor tissue by external AMF.

6.9 Conclusions

A computational modeling approach was applied for iron oxide MNPs to treat brain tumors. The pressure-induced nanofluid causes the deformation effect in the tumor. The back and forth motion of elastic tissue gives rise to the diffusion of nanofluid in the tumor. Stress causes strain and results in deformation displacement of brain tissue. The nanofluid's concentration and tumor temperature follow the Gaussian distribution in the brain tissue. Temperature-dependent blood perfusion increases in healthy tissue and decreases in cancerous tissue. The infusion pressure, infusion velocity, concentration, tumor temperature, and the fraction of tumor damage are maximum at the tumor center, and these decrease on moving from the center of the tumor to the radial outward direction. The maximum brain tumor is damaged with minimum collateral thermal damage. The comparison of the simulated results with preexisting literature further strengthens the present work. The parameters frequency and amplitude of AMF are sensitive to the heating effect. The increase or decrease in these parameters causes an increase or decrease in the cancerous tissue temperature. This work presents state-of-the-art treatment protocol for poroelastic brain tumor therapy which is directly applicable in clinical setting for cancer patients. The simulations offer cold test treatment as opposed to expending a lot of money on experimentation that is time-consuming. This work has also extensive applications in biomedical engineering for developing better, faster, and cost-efficient devices. Biomedical devices have paved the way to adopt mathematical methods based on simulations in the industry. It is believed that simulations can play a holistic part in the biomedical industry.

References

[1] Ferlay J, Soerjomataram I, Dikshit R, Eser S, Mathers C, Rebelo M, et al. Cancer incidence and mortality worldwide: sources, methods and major patterns in GLOBOCAN 2012. Int J Cancer 2015;136:E359–86.

[2] Jaroudi R, Baravdish G, Johansson BT, Åström F. Numerical reconstruction of brain tumours. Inverse Prob Sci Eng 2018;25:1–21.

[3] Louis DN, Perry A, Reifenberger G, von Deimling A, Figarella-Branger D, Cavenee WK, et al. The 2016 World Health Organization classification of tumors of the central nervous system: a summary. Acta Neuropathol 2016;131:803–20.

[4] Kleihues P, Burger PC, Scheithauer BW. The new WHO classification of brain tumours. Brain Pathol 1993;3:255–68.

[5] DeAngelis LM. Brain tumors. N Engl J Med 2001;344:114–23.

[6] Bernier J, Domenge C, Ozsahin M, Matuszewska K, Lefèbvre J-L, Greiner RH, et al. Postoperative irradiation with or without concomitant chemotherapy for locally advanced head and neck cancer. N Engl J Med 2004;350:1945–52.

[7] Wolff JE, Trilling T, MoÈlenkamp G, Egeler RM, JuÈrgens H. Chemosensitivity of glioma cells in vitro: a meta analysis. J Cancer Res Clin Oncol 1999;125:481–6.

[8] Pardridge WM. Drug targeting to the brain. Pharm Res 2007;24:1733–44.

[9] Pearson JR, Regad T. Targeting cellular pathways in glioblastoma multiforme. Signal Transduct Target Ther 2017;2:1–11.

[10] Pucci C, De Pasquale D, Marino A, Martinelli C, Lauciello S, Ciofani G. Hybrid magnetic nanovectors promote selective glioblastoma cell death through a combined effect of lysosomal membrane permeabilization and chemotherapy. ACS Appl Mater Interfaces 2020;12:29037–55.

[11] Nakagawa K, Aoki Y, Fujimaki T, Tago M, Terahara A, Karasawa K, et al. High-dose conformal radiotherapy influenced the pattern of failure but did not improve survival in glioblastoma multiforme. Int J Radiat Oncol Biol Phys 1998;40:1141–9.

[12] Lee SW, Fraass BA, Marsh LH, Herbort K, Gebarski SS, Martel MK, et al. Patterns of failure following high-dose 3-D conformal radiotherapy for high-grade astrocytomas: a quantitative dosimetric study. Int J Radiat Oncol Biol Phys 1999;43:79–88.

[13] Shaw E, Scott C, Souhami L, Dinapoli R, Kline R, Loeffler J, et al. Single dose radiosurgical treatment of recurrent previously irradiated primary brain tumors and brain metastases: final report of RTOG protocol 90-05. Int J Radiat Oncol Biol Phys 2000;47:291–8.

[14] Johannsen M, Gneveckow U, Eckelt L, Feussner A, Waldöfner N, Scholz R, et al. Clinical hyperthermia of prostate cancer using magnetic nanoparticles: presentation of a new interstitial technique. Int J Hyperth 2005;21:637–47.

[15] Christophi C, Winkworth A, Muralihdaran V, Evans P. The treatment of malignancy by hyperthermia. Surg Oncol 1998;7:83–90.

[16] Gilchrist R, Medal R, Shorey WD, Hanselman RC, Parrott JC, Taylor CB. Selective inductive heating of lymph nodes. Ann Surg 1957;146:596.

[17] Pizzichelli G, Di Michele F, Sinibaldi E. An analytical model for nanoparticles concentration resulting from infusion into poroelastic brain tissue. Math Biosci 2016;272:6–14.

[18] Di Michele F, Pizzichelli G, Mazzolai B, Sinibaldi E. On the preliminary design of hyperthermia treatments based on infusion and heating of magnetic nanofluids. Math Biosci 2015;262:105–16.

[19] Basser PJ. Interstitial pressure, volume, and flow during infusion into brain tissue. Microvasc Res 1992;44:143–65.

[20] Sobey I, Eisenträger A, Wirth B, Czosnyka M. Simulation of cerebral infusion tests using a poroelastic model. Int J Numer Anal Model B 2012;3:52–64.

[21] Su D, Ma R, Zhu L. Numerical study of nanofluid infusion in deformable tissues for hyperthermia cancer treatments. Med Biol Eng Comput 2011;49:1233–40.

[22] Lin C-T, Liu K-C. Estimation for the heating effect of magnetic nanoparticles in perfused tissues. Int Commun Heat Mass Transfer 2009;36:241–4.

[23] Wu W, Jiang C, Roy VA. Recent progress in magnetic iron oxide–semiconductor composite nanomaterials as promising photocatalysts. Nanoscale 2015;7:38–58.
[24] Laurent S, Dutz S, Häfeli UO, Mahmoudi M. Magnetic fluid hyperthermia: focus on superparamagnetic iron oxide nanoparticles. Adv Colloid Interf Sci 2011;166:8–23.
[25] Fatima H, Lee D-W, Yun HJ, Kim K-S. Shape-controlled synthesis of magnetic Fe_3O_4 nanoparticles with different iron precursors and capping agents. RSC Adv 2018;8:22917–23.
[26] Liu F, Cao P, Zhang H, Tian J, Xiao C, Shen C, et al. Novel nanopyramid arrays of magnetite. Adv Mater 2005;17:1893–7.
[27] Biot MA. General solutions of the equations of elasticity and consolidation for a porous material. J Appl Mech 1956;23:91–6.
[28] Biot M, Willis D. The elastic coeffcients of the theory of consolidation. J Appl Mech 1957;15:594–601.
[29] Biot MA. Theory of elasticity and consolidation for a porous anisotropic solid. J Appl Phys 1955;26:182–5.
[30] Makhnenko RY, Labuz JF. Elastic and inelastic deformation of fluid-saturated rock. Philos Trans R Soc A Math Phys Eng Sci 2016;374, 20150422.
[31] Chen X, Sarntinoranont M. Biphasic finite element model of solute transport for direct infusion into nervous tissue. Ann Biomed Eng 2007;35:2145–58.
[32] Netti PA, Baxter LT, Boucher Y, Skalak R, Jain RK. Macro-and microscopic fluid transport in living tissues: application to solid tumors. AIChE J 1997;43:818–34.
[33] Ganpule S, Daphalapurkar N, Cetingul M, Ramesh K. Effect of bulk modulus on deformation of the brain under rotational accelerations. Shock Waves 2018;28:127–39.
[34] Mackay DM, Freyberg D, Roberts P, Cherry J. A natural gradient experiment on solute transport in a sand aquifer: 1. Approach and overview of plume movement. Water Resour Res 1986;22:2017–29.
[35] Rosensweig RE. Heating magnetic fluid with alternating magnetic field. J Magn Magn Mater 2002;252:370–4.
[36] Javidi M, Heydari M, Karimi A, Haghpanahi M, Navidbakhsh M, Razmkon A. Evaluation of the effects of injection velocity and different gel concentrations on nanoparticles in hyperthermia therapy. J Biomed Phys Eng 2014;4:151.
[37] Rossmann C, Haemmerich D. Review of temperature dependence of thermal properties, dielectric properties, and perfusion of biological tissues at hyperthermic and ablation temperatures. Crit Rev Biomed Eng 2014;42:467–92.
[38] Pennes HH. Analysis of tissue and arterial blood temperatures in the resting human forearm. J Appl Physiol 1948;1:93–122.
[39] LeBrun A, Ma R, Zhu L. MicroCT image based simulation to design heating protocols in magnetic nanoparticle hyperthermia for cancer treatment. J Therm Biol 2016;62:129–37.
[40] Tompkinsn D, Vanderby R, Klein S, Beckman W, Steeves R, Frye D, et al. Temperature-dependent versus constant-rate blood perfusion modelling in ferromagnetic thermoseed hyperthermia: results with a model of the human prostate. Int J Hyperth 1994;10:517–36.
[41] Lang J, Erdmann B, Seebass M. Impact of nonlinear heat transfer on temperature control in regional hyperthermia. IEEE Trans Biomed Eng 1999;46:1129–38.
[42] Huang H-C, Rege K, Heys JJ. Spatiotemporal temperature distribution and cancer cell death in response to extracellular hyperthermia induced by gold nanorods. ACS Nano 2010;4:2892–900.
[43] Murbach M, Neufeld E, Capstick M, Kainz W, Brunner DO, Samaras T, et al. Thermal tissue damage model analyzed for different whole-body SAR and scan durations for standard MR body coils. Magn Reson Med 2014;71:421–31.
[44] Budday S, Nay R, de Rooij R, Steinmann P, Wyrobek T, Ovaert TC, et al. Mechanical properties of gray and white matter brain tissue by indentation. J Mech Behav Biomed Mater 2015;46:318–30.
[45] Comley K, Fleck N. Deep penetration and liquid injection into adipose tissue. J Mech Mater Struct 2011;6:127–40.
[46] Præstmark KA, Stallknecht B, Jensen ML, Sparre T, Madsen NB, Kildegaard J. Injection technique and pen needle design affect leakage from skin after subcutaneous injections. J Diabetes Sci Technol 2016;10:914–22.

CHAPTER 7

Finite element modeling analysis of hyperthermia of female breast cancer in three dimensions

The breast is generally known as the front part of the chest and physiologically termed as mammary glands. https://www.emedicinehealth.com/breast/article_em.htm#mammary_gland_design. It is a female breast tissue which is milk-producing organ that lies over the chest muscle. The milk-producing part consists of 15–20 lobes. The milk flows in the ducts to the outward skin called the nipple and the dark area surrounding the nipple is called the areola. Ligaments and connective tissues support the breast. Breast cancer develops exclusively in women as compared with men. Famous breast cancers include malignant, ductal carcinoma, lobular carcinoma, invasive ductal carcinoma, and breast fibroadenoma, https://www.webmd.com/women/picture-of-the-breasts#1. One out of eight US women is diagnosed with breast cancer, https://www.nationalbreastcancer.org/breast-cancer-facts with the visual clue shown in Fig. 7.1 below.

Breast cancer is a major cause of mortality worldwide. In the United States, in 2019, there were an estimated 268,600 breast cancer cases in women and 2670 cancer cases identified in men. From 2006 to 2015 female breast cancer cases increased by 0.4% per year and in 2019 an estimated 42,260 deaths occurred which include both male and female [1]. According to The World Health Organization, in 2005, an estimated 7.6 million people died of breast tumor and more than 70% of all cancer-related deaths happen in underdeveloped countries due to a lack of diagnosis and treatment facilities. Prominent symptoms of breast cancer are a lump in the breast, nipple retraction, asymmetry, blood-stained nipple discharge, eczematous, and skin retraction [2]. In 2008, 1,383,500 breast cancer cases and 458,400 cancer-related deaths were identified and half of these deaths were in third world countries [3]. The main risk factors for breast cancer are a family history of breast cancer, alcohol intake, physical inactivity, obesity, and smoking [4].

The MFH is better than the conventional noninvasive treatment techniques due to the generation of heat in deep-seated tumors with minimum normal tissue damage. Different researchers have attempted to treat breast cancer using MFH. The prominent approaches include the work by Miaskowski et al. [5] who used the magnetite MNPs to treat female breast

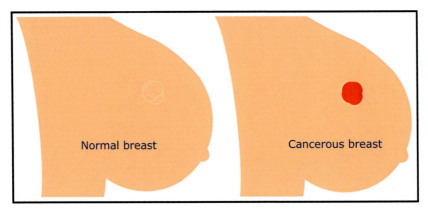

Fig. 7.1
Normal and cancerous female breast cups.

cancer. They proposed a theoretical formula based on specific absorption rate to determine the rise in temperature breast cancer. This formula agrees well with the experiments conducted on female breast cancer phantom. In another study [6], the author treated numerically the MFH of female breast cancer. They developed an artificial female breast phantom and transformed the experimental results on breast anatomy models. The study [7] dealt with the hyperthermia differently; the authors studied the recurrence of tumor in the chest wall experimentally by inserting probes at different locations in the recurrence region. The perfusion effect on the thermal map was investigated along with thermal conductivity through the solution of Penne's bioheat equation.

7.1 Physical properties of nanofluid

In the present study, we are considering the nanofluid of iron oxide (Fe_3O_4) MNPs with a size of 19nm. Octane is used as base fluid, which is generally used in hyperthermia studies. The density of these MNPs is ρ_p=5240kg/m^3 and that of the base fluid, octane is ρ_{bf}=698.6kg/m^3 [6,8]. The MNPs with size <100nm are suspended in the base fluids such as water, propylene glycol forms, or ethylene glycol [9]. The details of all calculations of properties of nanofluid that we will use in the current study can be found in Supplementary material: Appendix D.

7.2 Mathematical modeling formulation of the problem

7.2.1 Nanofluid infusion in the tumor

Nanofluid can be injected into the tumor [10] either intravenously or through needle approach [11,12]. We have applied the needle approach where nanofluid is administered in the tumor from needle tip following Darcy's Law demonstrated in Eq. (4.2). If the volumetric flow rate of nanofluid is 5μL/min, then the flux of nanofluid leaving the needle can be calculated using the formula (4.19) [13] as flux$_{nf}$=5.63×10^{-2} kg/(m² s) for $\dot{V}$=5μL/min, A_{needle}=π×(0.000686m²), and ρ_{np}=5240 kg/m³.

7.2.2 The diffusion of nanofluid in the tumor

After infusion, nanofluid starts to diffuse throughout tumor interstitium following diffusion model (4.4) where the diffusion coefficient D_i can be computed using the Stokes-Einstein model (4.5). Substituting the values of all parameters defined in Table 7.1, its value becomes 4.69×10^{-11} m²/s. Initially, concentration in all domains is zero. The mass concentration of the nanofluid flowing in the tumor is computed to be 354.17 kg/m³–1024.29 mol/m³ using model (4.20) with the values ϕ=0.2127 and ρ_{nf}=1665 kg/m³. The concentration at the outer boundary of the normal tissue is also taken zero.

7.2.3 Heat produced by Fe$_3$O$_4$ MNPs

The heat generated by MNPs due to externally applied magnetic field is modeled by the Rosensweig formulation [14] given by Eq. (3.27)

$$Q_{np} = \pi\mu_0 H_0^2 f \chi'' \tag{7.1}$$

where the details of all the calculations are given in Supplementary material: Appendix D. The heat generated is calculated as 3.33×10^5 W/m³. This amount of heat will be later added to the PBHTM.

Table 7.1 Parameters of heat generation model.

Parameter	Description	Values	Units	Source
D	Diameter of MNP	19	nm	[6]
r_p	Radius of MNP	9.5	nm	N/A
δ	Legend layer thickness	2	nm	[6]
H_0	Magnetic field intensity	12	kA/m	Tuneable
f_0	Frequency of magnetic field	150	kHz	[6]
M_d	Domain magnetization	4.46 × 10^5	kA/m	[8]
M_s	Saturation of magnetization	446	kA/m	[6]
k_B	Boltzmann constant	1.38 × 10^{-23}	J/K	[8]
μ_0	Permeability of free space	1.256 × 10^{-6}	H/m	[8]
K	Magnetic anisotropy constant	4.10 × 10^4	J/m³	[8]
η	Dynamic viscosity of nano fluid	9.27 × 10^{-4}	Pa s	Appendix A
ρ	Density of MNPs	5240	kg/m³	[8]

7.2.4 Heat transfer in the breast tissue

Heat transfer in the breast tissue can be predicted using PBHM [15] expressed by Eq. (4.8), where all variables associated with the model are defined with the model equations. We will predict the temperature profiles using this model. The temperature in the normal tissue is computed using the model (4.7) without Q_{np}. All the parameters contributing to the above model are defined in Table 7.2. The IC includes zero initial temperature and the BC includes convective BC where $h = 20\,\text{W/K/m}^2$ is the coefficient of heat transfer and T_{ext} is 37°C.

7.2.5 Prediction of the fraction of tumor necrosis

The fraction of tissue injury will be predicted using model [17] which is expressed by Eq. (4.11), where all the variables have been defined with the model and parameters included in the model are defined in Table 7.3.

7.3 Sensitivity analysis

The parameters involved in the electromagnetic heating are more sensitive. A minor fluctuation in the input may produce large output. The sensitivity coefficient S_i is defined as

$$S_i = \left(\frac{\partial Y}{\partial X_i}\right)\frac{X_i}{Y} \tag{7.2}$$

where the quotient X_i/Y is due to normalization which is done to avoid the role of units [19]. We will only investigate the sensitivity of frequency and amplitude of the applied magnetic field on tumor heating. We will also perform sensitivity analysis to investigate the impact of different mesh solutions of Eq. (4.8) on tumor heating.

Table 7.2 Breast gland parameters.

Parameter	Description	Values	Units	Source
T_b	Arterial blood temperature	310.15	K	[8]
ω_b	Blood perfusion rate	0.0067	1/s	[16]
Q_{met}	Metabolic heat	700	W/m^3	[16]
ρ_b	Density of blood	1058	kg/m^3	[16]
k	Thermal conductivity	0.33	W/m/K	[16]
c	Heat capacity	2960	J/kg/K	[16]

Table 7.3 Parameters used in the tumor damage model.

Parameter	Description	Cancer cells	Units	Source
A	Frequency factor	1.8×10^{36}	1/s	[18]
R	Universal gas constant	8.23	J/mol/K	[18]
E_a	Activation energy	2.38×10^5	J/mol	[18]

7.4 The AMF generated by the coil

The current-carrying coil generates a magnetic field given as

$$\nabla \times \boldsymbol{H} = \boldsymbol{J}_e,$$
$$\boldsymbol{B} = \nabla \times \boldsymbol{A} \tag{7.3}$$

associated with Ampere's law

$$\nabla \times \left(\frac{1}{\mu_0 \mu_r}\boldsymbol{B}\right) - \sigma \boldsymbol{v} \times \boldsymbol{B} = \boldsymbol{J}_e,$$
$$\boldsymbol{B} = \nabla \times \boldsymbol{A} \tag{7.4}$$

where magnetic and electric fields are linked as

$$\boldsymbol{B} = \mu_0 \mu_r \boldsymbol{H},$$
$$\boldsymbol{D} = \varepsilon_0 \varepsilon_r \boldsymbol{E} \tag{7.5}$$

the magnetic insulation is given by

$$\boldsymbol{n} \times \boldsymbol{A} = 0 \tag{7.6}$$

and initially, $\boldsymbol{A} = (0, 0, 0)$ Wb/m. The coil current flowing in the conductor is given by

$$I_{\text{coil}} = \int_{\partial \Omega} \boldsymbol{J} \cdot \boldsymbol{n} \tag{7.7}$$

For the frequency domain, AMF is given by.

$$(j\omega\sigma - \omega^2 \varepsilon_0 \varepsilon_r)\boldsymbol{A} + \nabla \times \boldsymbol{H} = \boldsymbol{J}_e,$$
$$\boldsymbol{B} = \nabla \times \boldsymbol{A} \tag{7.8}$$

where associated Ampere's law is expressed by.

$$(j\omega\sigma - \omega^2 \varepsilon_0 \varepsilon_r)\boldsymbol{A} + \nabla \times \left(\frac{1}{\mu_0 \mu_r}\boldsymbol{B}\right) - \sigma \boldsymbol{v} \times \boldsymbol{B} = \boldsymbol{J}_e,$$
$$\boldsymbol{B} = \nabla \times \boldsymbol{A} \tag{7.9}$$

where μ_r is relative permeability, σ is electrical conductivity, ω is the angular frequency, ε_r is relative permittivity, and j is the current density.

7.5 Results

For the implementation of our problem of hyperthermia processes on COMSOL Multiphysics, we proceed as follows: From the model wizard, 3D space dimension was added. Darcy's law from the "Porous media and subsurface flow" node was added for the infusion of nanofluid in the tumor. We have added a convection-diffusion equation from the "transport of diluted species" node which is selected from the "Chemical species transport" node for the nanofluid diffusion in the tumor interstitium. For the transfer of heat in the breast tissue, we have added a "bioheat equation." The study for infusion model is added as a steady-state while for all the remaining physics was added as time-dependent. The 3D geometry of the breast cup is constructed as follows: a tumor with a radius of 10mm was constructed with normal tissue of radius 30mm around this tumor. A 15-gauge needle with an outer diameter 1.83mm, inner diameter 1.732mm, and a wall of thickness 0.229mm was used. The final geometry is shown in Fig. 7.2. We added the muscle as the material for tumor and normal tissues while that for injecting needle is added as a steel AISI 4340. The parameters were substituted from Tables 7.1–7.3, and Supplementary material: Appendix A. The ICs and BCs were added following their respective sections.

The mesh of the model is generated in an extra-fine mode, as demonstrated in Fig. 7.3.

Firstly, we have simulated the velocity of nanofluid as shown in Fig. 7.4A. Maximum velocity of 55.9 μm/s was obtained at the needle tip. To predict velocity quantitatively L1, a cutline 3D, is drawn as shown in Fig. 7.6B. The plot of velocity vs y-coordinate is demonstrated in

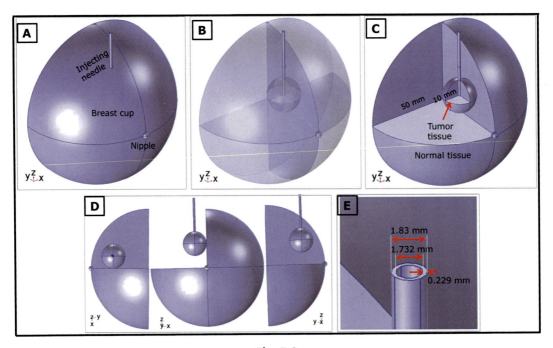

Fig. 7.2
Geometry construction of problem: (A) the injected needle in breast cup, (B) breast cup with transparent view, (C) model without fourth quadrant, (D) model view in *XY*, *YZ*, and *ZX* planes, and (E) dimensions of the injected needle.

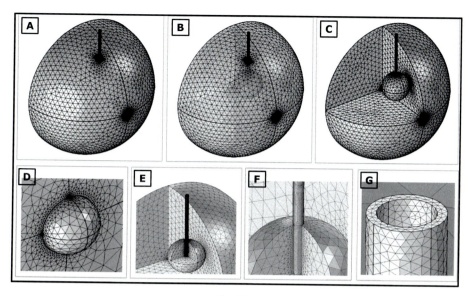

Fig. 7.3
Meshing the model: (A) mesh has 305,868 tetrahedral domain, 2641 edge, and 42,159 boundary elements. Maximum element size is 3.85 mm and minimum of 0.165 mm. The narrow region has a resolution of 0.85, the growth rate of the maximum element was 1.35, and curvature factor was 0.3. (B) Mesh model in transparent view. (C) Mesh model in the absence of fourth quadrant. (D) Zoomed nipple of breast cup. (E) Both normal and tumor tissues without fourth quadrant. (F) Zoomed injected needle. (G) Zoomed cross section of the needle.

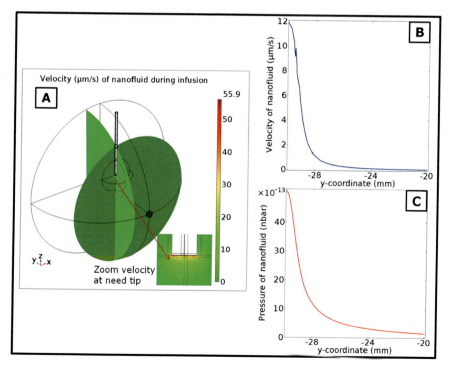

Fig. 7.4
Nanofluid injection in the tumor: (A) 3D velocity of nanofluid in the breast cup. (B) Velocity of nanofluid vs y-coordinate. (C) Pressure of nanofluid vs y-coordinate.

Fig. 7.4B. The obtained graph was symmetrical about a line $y=-30$ mm in Gaussian distribution form. The peak value of the velocity was 12 μm/s and if the line segment L1 was drawn more closely to the needle tip, the maximum value reached 55.9 μm/s. The pressure variation of nanofluid is shown in Fig. 7.4C along the same line segment L1. The pressure distribution is also in Gaussian form and is not steeper like the velocity curve. Maximum pressure of 49×10^{-13} nbar was obtained and it decreases on moving from the center of the tumor to the outer boundary of normal tissue.

When a nanofluid is injected into the tumor, it pushes the breast tissue back and tries to escape through the tissue wall and needle interface. Through this gap nanofluid leaks and generates backflow. It is modeled by the Navier-Stokes equation (4.2) along with ICs and BCs. The simulation of backflow is shown in Fig. 7.5A. The backflow is represented by streamlines of nanofluid velocity. The streamlines with a zoomed view near the needle tip are demonstrated in Fig. 7.5B where the backflow is apparent along with the needle interface. The backflow is also highlighted by the streamlines in Fig. 7.5C.

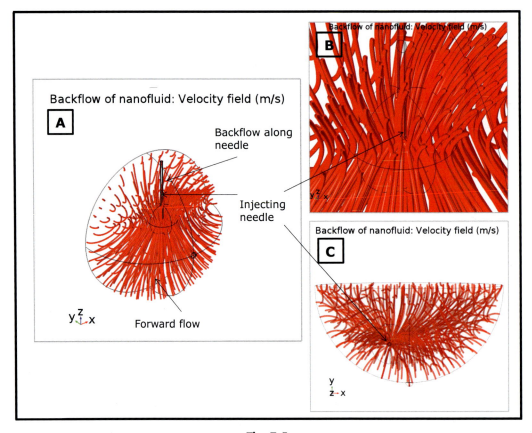

Fig. 7.5

Simulation of the backflow velocity: (A) 3D velocity of backflow, (B) velocity at the needle tip, and (C) velocity in *XY*-plane.

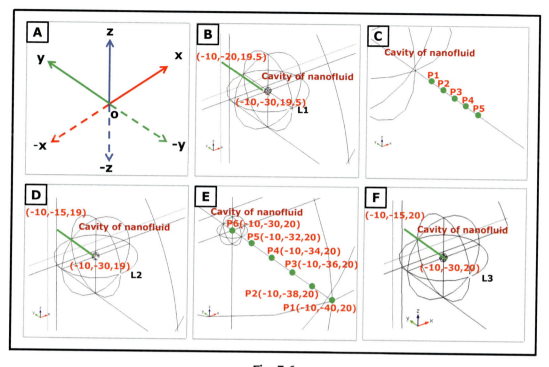

Fig. 7.6

Selected points and line segments with visual representation: (A) Cartesian coordinates system, (B) L1, cutline 3D, (C) selected points for concentration estimation, (D) L2, cutline 3D, (E) selected points for temperature and fraction of tissue necrosis estimation, and (F) L3, cutline 3D.

After the nanofluid infusion, the needle is taken out and the injected nanofluid forms a cavity at the center of the tumor. We assumed that the nanofluid forms a spherical cavity. The pressure induced-nanofluid diffuses in the tumor interstitium according to the convection-diffusion equation. The time-dependent concentration of nanofluid is simulated after 24h which is demonstrated in Fig. 7.7A. Nanofluid flows outside from the center of the tumor with a mass concentration of 1024.29 mol/m^3. We have selected points P_i: $(-10, i = [-31.2:0.2:-32], 20)$ mm in breast tissue for quantitative analysis as depicted in Fig. 7.6C. The concentration against time profile is demonstrated in Fig. 7.7B. As the concentration at point P_1 is larger than that at point P_5, the concentration at the tumor center is maximum as compared to the concentration at the boundary of body tissue. A line segment L2 is drawn to plot concentration against the y-axis as shown in Fig. 7.6D. At times $t=[0:1:5]$ h along with L2, the concentration is symmetrical about the y-axis as demonstrated in Fig. 7.7C. The results show that with time the concentration profiles shift to higher values. The concentration is higher at the tumor center and vanishes beyond the outer boundary of the body tissue.

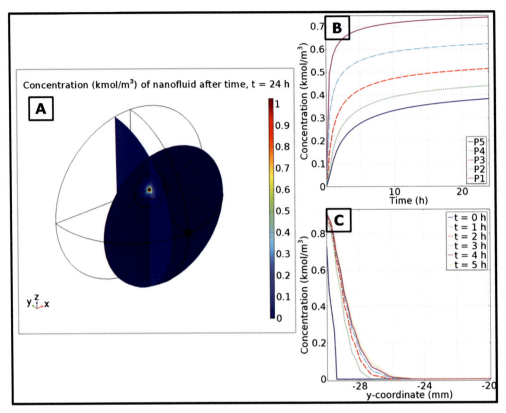

Fig. 7.7
Simulation of the diffusion model: (A) 3D distribution of concentration in the breast tissue, (B) concentration vs time at selected points, and (C) concentration vs y-axis at selected times.

The concentration vs y-axis profiles follow Gaussian distribution and therefore are symmetrical about the y-axis. Being symmetrical, we have shown only half parts of the graphs. Our simulations agree well with the analytical solution [20] for concentration as shown in Fig. 7.8 and the analytical solution is expressed as.

$$C = C_i + \left(\frac{M_0}{4\pi D_i t}\right) e^{-\left(\frac{r^2}{4D_i t}\right)} \tag{7.10}$$

where C_i is the initial concentration, t is time, M_0 is the adjustable constants, r is the radial distance from the point source, and D_i is the diffusion coefficient.

Simulation of the diffusive flux of the nanofluid with arrow plots is demonstrated in Fig. 7.9A. Transient analysis for diffusive flux at specific points P_1 to P_5 are shown in Fig. 7.9B. The selected points are visually shown in Fig. 7.6C. The diffusive flux varies from a maximum value at point P_1 to the minimum at point P_5. The diffusive flux near the cavity is exponentially

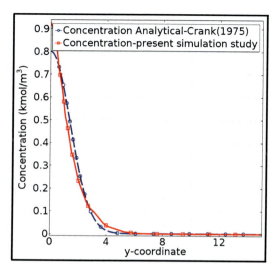

Fig. 7.8
Validation of simulations with an analytical solution for concentration.

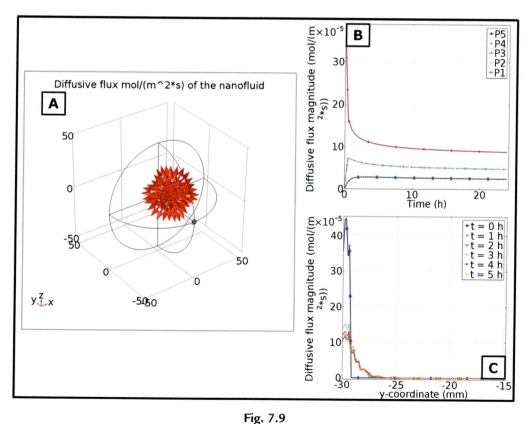

Fig. 7.9
Diffusive flux of nanofluid: (A) 3D diffusive flux distribution, (B) diffusive flux against time at selected points, and (C) diffusive flux against y-axis at selected times.

decaying and beyond the cavity, it increases first and after reaching a peak value it again decreases to the minimum value. The results show that initially diffusive flux was maximum and at time 0–5 h, it attenuated toward a minimum value.

After diffusion, the external magnetic field is switched on which induced vibrations in MNPs. Heat is released under Neel and Brownian relaxation effects. Heat transfer is modeled through the bioheat model (4.8) in tumor and normal tissues with Q_{np} and without the terms Q_{np}. The 3D distribution of temperature in the breast tissue after 60 min is shown in Fig. 7.10A. In the first 10 min of heating, the temperature rises to 46.8°C inside the tumor from a normal tissue temperature of 37°C and it remains in a stationary state till the end of heating time. To analyze the temperature quantitatively, we have selected points $P_i = (-10, [-40:2:-30], 20)$ that are visualized in Fig. 7.6E. The temperature against time curves at the selected points are simulated in Fig. 7.10B. The temperature near the tumor tissue is higher than the temperature near the outer boundary of the tumor. The temperature against the y-axis along with L3 at the selected times $t = [0:1:6]$ min is shown in Fig. 7.10C and L3 is visualized in Fig. 7.6F. The behavior of the temperature curves is identical to the Gaussian distribution curve and these curves move to the higher temperature with the elapse of time.

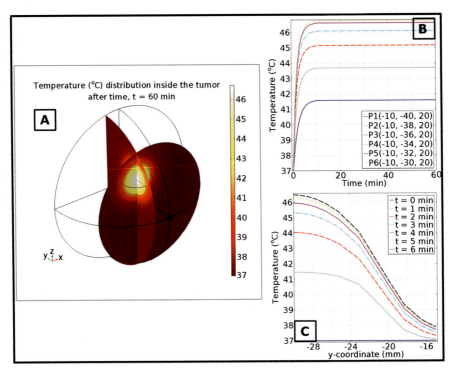

Fig. 7.10

Simulation of temperature distribution in the breast cup: (A) the 3D distribution of temperature, (B) temperature vs time plots at selected points, and (C) temperature against y-axis at selected times.

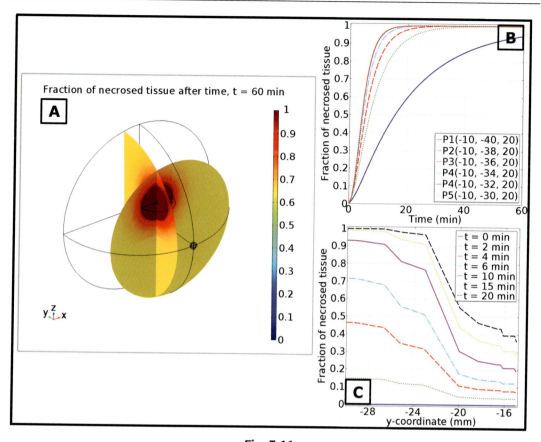

Fig. 7.11
Simulation of the fraction of tumor damage: (A) 3D tissue necrosis, (B) fraction of tissue damage vs time plots, and (C) fraction of tissue damage vs y-axis.

The elevated temperature developed due to the applied magnetic field is sustained to damage the tumor. The estimation of the fraction of tissue necrosis is simulated in Fig. 7.11A. Tissue necrosis is maximum at the center and minimum at the outer boundary of the tumor. The fraction of tissue damage vs time at selected points is shown in Fig. 7.11B and the selected points are visualized in Fig. 7.6E. The fraction of the tumor damage is 1 at point P_5 and this fraction is 0.95 at point P_1. These results show that more tumor is damaged near the center of the tumor than at the outer boundary of the tumor. The fraction of tissue necrosis against the y-axis at selected times is shown in Fig. 7.11C and the visual clue of L3 is shown in Fig. 7.6F. With time, the tissue damaged plots are shifted to higher values. Thus, maximum tumor necrosis is obtained at the maximum heating time.

We have validated our simulation with that of Miaskowski and Sawicki [6]. It was an identical experimental study performed on artificial phantoms of breast cups. They estimated the temperature against time profiles at the frequency $f = 150$ kHz. We have also predicted the

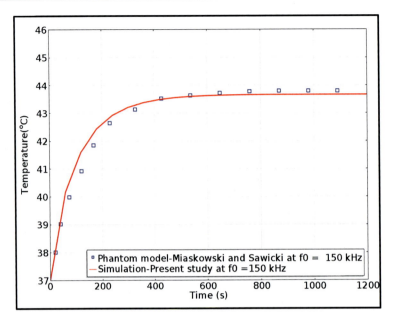

Fig. 7.12
Validation of simulation with experimental work.

temperature vs time curves at the frequency $f=150$ kHz through computer-based simulations at a tunable amplitude of AMF. Validation of simulation with experimental results is demonstrated in Fig. 7.12. Both curves agree well. It is evident that our simulation therapy works well.

In the current study, each parameter is much sensitive, a small change may produce a large fluctuation in output. We have investigated the sensitivity of amplitude and frequency of AMF. The impact of variation in amplitudes $H_0=10:1:15$ kA/m and frequency $f_0=20, 40, 60, 100, 200$ kHz on heating effect is demonstrated in Fig. 7.13. The tumor heating increases with increase in amplitudes and frequency. The simulation results show that the temperature of the tumor increases with increase in either the amplitude or frequency of the AMF.

Next, we have performed mesh-dependent analysis for the solution of PBHTM (4.8). We have investigated the impact of coarser, coarse, normal, fine, and finer meshes on this model, and results are shown in Fig. 7.14. The details about different meshes are demonstrated in Table 7.4. The results show that the finer is the mesh, the higher is the temperature through a minor fraction.

The heat by the MNPs is generated due to AMF crossing the breast cup. The AMF is developed by the coil conductors and is shown in Fig. 7.15. The two copper coil conductors were constructed surrounding the breast cup as shown in Fig. 7.15A. The conductors and breast cup are placed in a cube filled with air. The fine mesh of the model was generated as shown in

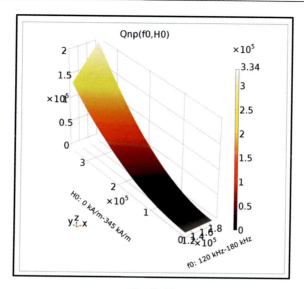

Fig. 7.13

Impact of the sensitivity of amplitude H_0 and frequency f_0 AMF on heating effect.

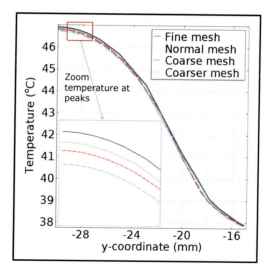

Fig. 7.14

Mesh-dependent solution of PBHTM.

Table 7.4 Meshing details.

Mesh type	Solution time	No. of the degree of freedom	Plus internal DOFs
Fine	137 s	54,548	30,968
Normal	86 s	36,967	26,512
Coarse	68 s	28,467	25,508
Coarser	50 s	18,719	20,028

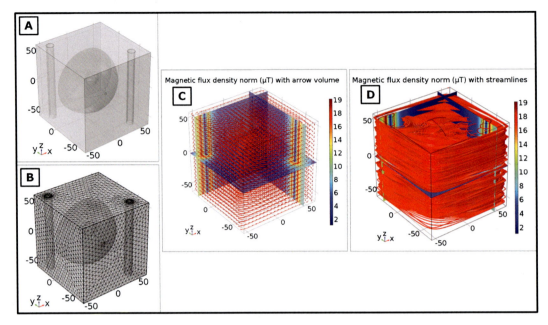

Fig. 7.15
Simulation of magnetic induction problem: (A) model geometry, a breast cup surrounded by coil conductors and air cube, (B) fine mesh of the problem, (C) arrow plot representation of magnetic flux density, and (D) streamlines representing magnetic flux density.

Fig. 7.15B. The magnetic flux density developed by the conductors is simulated by an arrow plot. The circular trend of the arrow plot around the breast cup is shown in Fig. 7.15C. The maximum value of magnetic flux density was obtained at 19 μT. The magnetic flux density in the form of streamlines was simulated in Fig. 7.15D. The streamline plot in XY-plane is shown in Fig. 7.16A. The magnetic lines of forces cross with the breast cup situated between the two coil conductors and these will induce oscillations in the MNPs. As a result of vibrations in MNPs, it releases heat that kills tumor cells. The heating of the tumor is simulated in Fig. 7.16B for transient analysis where the maximum temperature is 45°C. Lastly, we have simulated the core parameters of coil conductions as shown in Fig. 7.17. The coil potential, induced current density, current density norm, electric field (volume), electric field (streamline), and an electric field (XY-plane streamlines) are shown in Fig. 7.17A–F respectively.

Finite element modeling analysis of breast hyperthermia   111

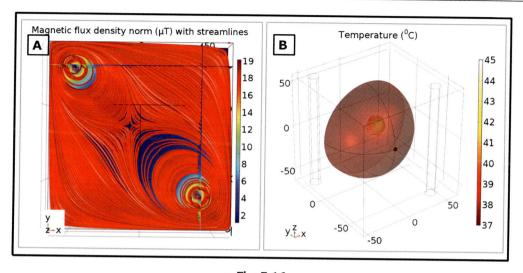

Fig. 7.16
(A) Streamline plot in XY-plane and (B) AMF developed the temperature distribution in the tumor.

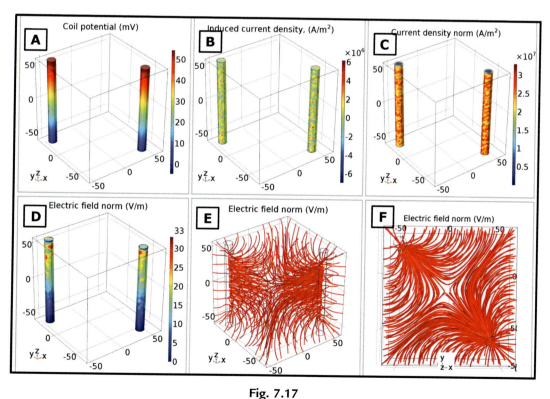

Fig. 7.17
Simulation of core parameters of coil: (A) potential of the coil, (B) induced current density, (C) norm of the current density, (D) electric field (volume), (E) electric field (streamline), and (F) electric field (XY-plane streamlines).

7.6 Conclusions

A 3D computational study of MFH of the breast tumors is performed and analyzed quantitatively. The injection of nanofluid with higher pressure will cause a backflow problem, therefore it is recommended that nanofluid should be infused at a slow rate. Tumor heating depends on MFD generated by the current-carrying coil, which ultimately depends on the frequency and amplitude of AMF. The breast tumor is damaged with minimum collateral thermal destruction. The amplitude and frequency of AMF are directly proportional to the increase in temperature. The more finer is the mesh, the higher will be the temperature. The infusion velocity, concentration, and temperature distribution are maximum at the center of the tumor and minimum at the outer boundary of the tumor. The temperature of the tumor elevated with increasing heating time. Our simulation results agree well with an identical experimental study.

References

[1] Gaugler J, James B, Johnson T, Marin A, Weuve J. 2019 Alzheimer's disease facts and figures. Alzheimers Dement 2019;15:321–87.
[2] World Health Organization. Cancer control: Knowledge into action. WHO guide for effective programmes: prevention. World Health Organization; 2007.
[3] Ferlay J, Shin H, Bray F, Forman D, Mathers C, Parkin D. Cancer incidence and mortality worldwide IARC cancer base 2008. Lyon, France: International Agency for Research on Cancer; 2008.
[4] Surdyka JA, Surdyka D, Stanislawek A, Staroslawska E, Patyra KI. Selected breast cancer risk factors and early detection of the neoplasm in women from Lublin region attending screening program in St. John's Cancer Center, years 2005–2006. Ann Agric Environ Med 2014;21.
[5] Miaskowski A, Sawicki B, Krawczyk A, Yamada S. The application of magnetic fluid hyperthermia to breast cancer treatment. Electr Rev 2010;86:99–101.
[6] Miaskowski A, Sawicki B. Magnetic fluid hyperthermia modeling based on phantom measurements and realistic breast model. IEEE Trans Biomed Eng 2013;60:1806–13.
[7] Guiot C, Madon E, Allegro D, Pianta P, Baiotto B, Gabriele P. Perfusion and thermal field during hyperthermia. Experimental measurements and modelling in recurrent breast cancer. Phys Med Biol 1998;43:2831.
[8] Javidi M, Heydari M, Karimi A, Haghpanahi M, Navidbakhsh M, Razmkon A. Evaluation of the effects of injection velocity and different gel concentrations on nanoparticles in hyperthermia therapy. J Biomed Phys Eng 2014;4:151.
[9] Adhikary K, Banerjee M. A thermofluid analysis of the magnetic nanoparticles enhanced heating effects in tissues embedded with large blood vessel during magnetic fluid hyperthermia. J Nanopart 2016;2016, 6309231.
[10] Hassanpour S, Saboonchi A. Interstitial hyperthermia treatment of countercurrent vascular tissue: a comparison of Pennes, WJ and porous media bioheat models. J Therm Biol 2014;46:47–55.
[11] Salloum M, Ma R, Weeks D, Zhu L. Controlling nanoparticle delivery in magnetic nanoparticle hyperthermia for cancer treatment: experimental study in agarose gel. Int J Hyperth 2008;24:337–45.
[12] Salloum M, Ma R, Zhu L. An in-vivo experimental study of temperature elevations in animal tissue during magnetic nanoparticle hyperthermia. Int J Hyperth 2008;24:589–601.
[13] Di Michele F, Pizzichelli G, Mazzolai B, Sinibaldi E. On the preliminary design of hyperthermia treatments based on infusion and heating of magnetic nanofluids. Math Biosci 2015;262:105–16.

[14] Rosensweig RE. Heating magnetic fluid with alternating magnetic field. J Magn Magn Mater 2002;252:370–4.
[15] Pennes HH. Analysis of tissue and arterial blood temperatures in the resting human forearm. J Appl Physiol 1948;1:93–122.
[16] Hasgall P. ITIS database for thermal and electromagnetic parameters of biological tissues, Version 2.2, July 11th; 2012.
[17] Wang H, Wu J, Zhuo Z, Tang J. A three-dimensional model and numerical simulation regarding thermoseed mediated magnetic induction therapy conformal hyperthermia. Technol Health Care 2016;24:S827–39.
[18] LeBrun A, Ma R, Zhu L. MicroCT image based simulation to design heating protocols in magnetic nanoparticle hyperthermia for cancer treatment. J Therm Biol 2016;62:129–37.
[19] Atherton R, Schainker R, Ducot E. On the statistical sensitivity analysis of models for chemical kinetics. AIChE J 1975;21:441–8.
[20] Crank J. The mathematics of diffusion. Oxford University Press; 1979.

CHAPTER 8

Mathematical modeling and simulation of enhanced permeation and retention (EPR) effect with thermal analysis

In MFH, generally, two approaches are used to infuse MNPs in the tumor. In the first approach, MNPs are injected intravenously following the EPR effect. The MNPs enter the tumor vasculature through a leaky blood vessel and epithelial cell spacing [1]. In the second approach, MNPs are injected by intertumoral infusion or convection-enhanced delivery using needles of varying gauge sizes [2]. But this technique may not prove useful for the deep sited tumors and solid tumors where it may produce cracks in the tumor [3]. This approach is generally applied to inject the MNPs in the liver tumor [4], breast tumor [5], and tumors with irregular shape with multiple injection technique [6].

To deliver MNPs into the tumor is a critical problem. The MNPs reach tumor interstitium through extravasation from the tumor vessels supported by the EPR effect [7]. This distribution is heterogeneous and covers the surrounding region of the tumor [8]. The diffusion of MNPs in the tumor is a complex problem and depends on the injection pressure [9]. The MNPs are of the size of the naturally occurring biological molecules that allows them to be used in the biological phenomenon. Their nanosize allows them to interact with biological molecules and to internalize into cells and cause them to respond either dynamically or selectively.

Under the EPR effect, after reaching the tumor, MNPs remain there. This effect is known as the "gold-standard" in the planning of the latest anticancer techniques. The EPR effect is an aggregation of leaky blood vessels due to angiogenic regulators, interstitial space between endothelial cells, and lymphatic drainage in the tumor. The tumor has leaky vasculature that permits MNPs to penetrate through epithelial cell gaps of sizes close to 4μm to reach interstitial tumor fluid [10]. We have proposed a diagram of the EPR effect as shown in Fig. 8.1, for which we will later build the computation theory to simulate. We in this research will investigate the EPR effect from the modeling and simulation approach. The Navier-Stokes equation coupled

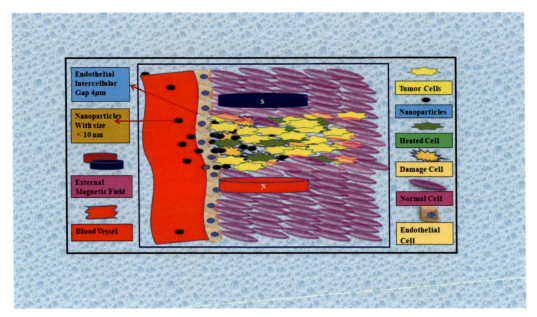

Fig. 8.1
Schematic diagram of enhanced permeation and retention effect (EPR).

with the continuity equation will be utilized to study the velocity of nanofluid flowing in the blood vessel. The transport of nanofluid in the porous tumor will be modeled by the convection-diffusion equation and this model will be simulated for the concentration of nanofluid in the porous tumor structure. Heat transfer in the porous tissue will be modeled by Penne's bioheat transfer model. We will analyze their FEM models for quantitative information. We will also perform the mesh-dependent solution of the Navier-Stokes equation for the velocity of the nanofluid in the blood vessel.

8.1 Physical properties of nanofluid

In this research, we have used nanofluid comprised of iron oxide Fe_3O_4 MNPs of size 10nm with a TEM image shown in Fig. 8.2 [11,12]. The density of MNPs is $\rho_p=5240 \text{kgm}^{-3}$ and of base fluid is $\rho_{bf}=698.6 \text{ kg m}^{-3}$ [13]. The volume fraction of the nanofluid using Eq. (4.14) with $m_p=159.687$ g/mol, $m_{bf}=18.02$ g/mol becomes $\phi=0.6943$. The molar mass of nanofluid is $m_{nf}=177.71$ g/mol $\approx$ 0.1777 kg/mol. The effective density of nanofluid using Eq. (4.15) is $\rho_{nf}=3006 \text{ kg/m}^3$. The specific heat capacity of the MNPs and base fluids are $c_p=765$ J/kg/K and $c_{nf}=4183$ J/kg/K, respectively. The effective heat capacity of the nanofluid using Eq. (4.16) becomes $c=1809.79$ J/kg/K. The nanofluid's thermal conductivity using Eq. (4.17) with $n=3$ for MNPs in 3D, and thermal conductivities of the base fluid and MNPs are $k_{bf}=0.6065$ W/m/K and $k_{np}=30$ W/m/K,

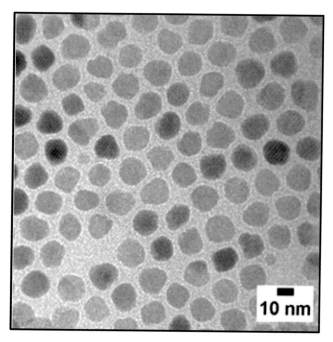

Fig. 8.2
TEM image of Fe_3O_4 nanoparticles in deionized water.

respectively, becomes $k_{nf}=4.043$ W/m/K. The viscosity of nanofluid using Eq. (4.18) is 0.01722 Pa s, since the viscosity of the base fluid is 8.90×10^{-4} Pa s.

8.2 Mathematical modeling formulation of the problem

8.2.1 Nanofluid flow in the blood vessel

Nanofluid flow in the blood vessel is modeled through the Navier-Stokes equation coupled with the continuity equation (4.1). Where ρ_{nf} is the density of the nanofluid and η is the dynamic viscosity of the nanofluid. The IC includes both the velocity and pressure being zero in the blood vessel as demonstrated below

$$u = 0, p = 0 \tag{8.1}$$

The BC include that the inlet is

$$u = -U_0 n \tag{8.2}$$

where U_0 is the inflow velocity of the nanofluid in the blood vessel that can be calculated using the expression

$$U_0 = Q/A \tag{8.3}$$

where Q is the flow rate of nanofluid at the inlet which we ae taking 3 µL/min and A is the area of the cross-section for the blood vessel which is calculated to be 5.03×10^{-11} m^2 for the blood vessel with the radius 4 µm. The inflow velocity at the inlet becomes 9.95×10^{-1} m/s. And the outlet is defined as

$$-p\mathbf{I} + \eta\left(\nabla \mathbf{u} + (\nabla \mathbf{u})^T\right)n = -\hat{p}_0 n, \quad \hat{p}_0 \leq p_0 \tag{8.4}$$

8.2.2 Diffusion of nanoflow in the tumor interstitium

The diffusion of nanofluid in the porous tumor is modeled through the convection-diffusion equation (4.4). We are considering only the convection enhanced diffusion of the nanofluid and neglecting the microscale interactions of nanofluid with the tumor matrix while flowing through it. The D^k is the diffusion coefficient that can be calculated by using the Stokes-Einstein equation (4.5). Where $k_B = 1.38 \times 10^{-23}$ J/K is Boltzmann constant, $T = 310.15$ K is absolute temperature, $\eta_{nf} = 0.01722$ Pa s is the viscosity of nanofluid, and $r_p = 7.5$ nm is the radius of a nanoparticle. Using these values, D^k is calculated to be 5.94×10^{-11} m^2/s, The IC includes zero initial concentration in the whole domain

$$c^k = 0 \tag{8.5}$$

and BC includes no flux at the outer boundary of the tissue

$$-n \cdot \mathbf{N}^k = 0 \tag{8.6}$$

8.2.3 Heat transfer in the porous tumor interstitium

We are considering the tumor of the breast gland in this study where the properties of breast organs are listed in Table 8.1. We will employ PBHTM [16] to study the transfer of heat in the tumor tissue. We consider an ideal distribution during the diffusion of MNPs in the tumor

Table 8.1 Breast gland parameters.

Parameter	Description	Values	Units	Source
T_b	Arterial blood temperature	310.15	K	[14]
ω_b	Blood perfusion rate	0.0067	s^{-1}	[15]
Q_{met}	Metabolic heat	700	W m^{-3}	[15]
ρ_b	Density of blood	1058	kg m^{-3}	[15]
k	Thermal conductivity	0.33	W m^{-1}K^{-1}	[15]
c	Heat capacity	2960	J kg^{-1}K^{-1}	[15]

Table 8.2 Parameters of heat generation model.

Parameter	Description	Values	Units	Source
D	Diameter of MNP	10	nm	[14]
r_p	Radius of MNP	5	nm	N/A
δ	Legend layer thickness	2	nm	[18]
H_0	Magnetic field intensity	12	kA m^{-1}	Adjustable
f_0	Frequency of magnetic field	150	kHz	[18]
M_d	Domain magnetization	4.46×10^8	kA m^{-1}	[14]
M_s	Saturation of magnetization	4.46×10^2	kA m^{-1}	[18]
k_B	Boltzmann constant	1.38×10^{-23}	J K^{-1}	[14]
μ_0	Permeability of free space	1.256×10^{-6}	H m^{-1}	[14]
K	Magnetic anisotropy constant	4.10×10^4	J m^{-3}	[14]
ρ_p	Density of MNPs	5240	kg m^{-3}	[14]

before the heating effect. The heat transfer is formulated by Eq. (4.8) where ρ is tumor tissue density, c tumor tissue-specific heat, k is tumor tissue-specific thermal conductivity, T is tumor tissue temperature, ρ_b is blood density, ω_b is local blood perfusion rate, T_b is local arterial blood temperature, c_b blood specific heat, Q_m is metabolic heat generation rate, and Q_{np} is heat generated by MNPs and it is calculated as $Q_{np} = 3.32 \times 10^5$ W m^{-3} using R.E. Rosensweig formulation [17]. The values of all the parameters involved are tabulated in Table 8.2. The details of all calculations are given in Appendix E: supplementary material. The IC is given by $T = 310.15$ K in both tumors and healthy tissues. The first BCs include $n \cdot (-k\nabla T) = 0$ thermal insulation and convective boundary condition $-n \cdot (-k\nabla T) = h(T_{ext} - T)$ taken on the external boundary of the breast tumor. In this BC, $h = 200$ W K^{-1} m^{-2} represents heat transfer coefficient and $T_{ext} = 310.15$ K.

8.3 Results and discussions

We have constructed an artificial geometry of the EPR effect on COMSOL Multiphysics. A blood vessel of diameter 8 μm was constructed. Epithelial cells with a semimajor axis of 13 μm and a semiminor axis of 12 μm were created. Cancer cells of size 7 μm were generated using arrays. The whole geometry is shown in Fig. 8.3. The physics for the nanofluid flow in the blood vessels is selected as *Laminar flow*. For nanofluid diffusion in the tumor interstitium, the physics of the *Convection-diffusion equation* is added. The studies for *Laminar flow* and *Convection-diffusion equation* were selected as stationary and time-dependent respectively. Material for blood vessel and tumor were selected as water/liquid and bioheat/liver respectively. The ICs and BCs for both physics are added following their respective sections. The value of the diffusion coefficient was inserted from Eq. (4.5) for Fe_3O_4 magnetite MNPs of diameter 15 nm.

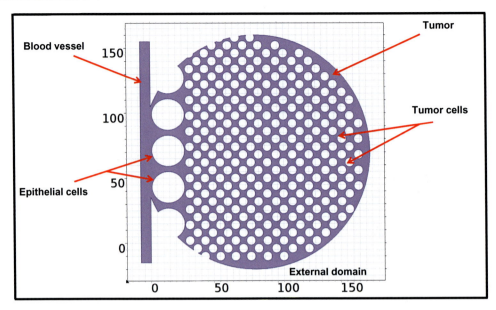

Fig. 8.3
The geometry of the problem: blood vessel, epithelial cells, and porous tumor.

After constructing geometry, adding physics, adding studies, materials, ICs, and BCs the mesh of the problem was generated as shown in Fig. 8.4. Where the details about this mesh are described in the caption.

After mesh generation the problem was solved for the velocity of nanofluid in the blood vessel and the surface plot is shown in Fig. 8.5A. The number of degrees of freedom solved was 204,048 and solution time was $t=48$ s. The maximum velocity achieved is 1.5 m/s. The zoomed plot for this simulation is shown in Fig. 8.5B. The simulation shows that during nanofluid flow in the blood vessels, nanofluid also penetrates the tumor interstitium through the spacing between epithelial cells. To investigate the behavior of velocity quantitatively, we have selected three horizontal line segments L1, L2, and L3 and three vertical line segments L4, L5, and L6 as shown in Fig. 8.5C. The corresponding simulations for velocity along horizontal line segments are shown in Fig. 8.5D. The velocity behavior along L1 is in parabolic shape and extends from 0 to 8 μm. This is the velocity in the blood vessels and is maximum at the center of the blood vessel and minimum near the walls of the blood vessels. A similar behavior is also predicted for velocity along line segment L3. The behavior of velocity along line segment L2 is also in parabolic shape extending from 0 to 16 μm but after this, velocity is attenuated with a small amplitude as compared to the previous one. This fluctuation continues until the curve gets a steady state through the cellular spacing of the tumor. This simulation shows the diffusion of nanofluid from blood vessel to tumor interstitium which is evident from the extension of parabolic shape beyond 8 μm which is the diameter of the blood vessels. These simulations also

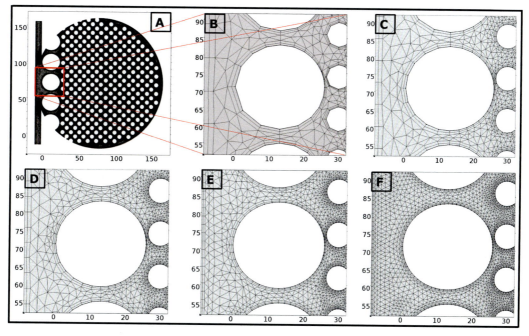

Fig. 8.4

Mesh generation of the problem: (A) extremely fine mesh of the whole problem: complete mesh consists of 106,936 domain and 9896 boundary elements, (B) zoomed extremely coarse mesh: complete mesh consists of 14,554 domain and 3172 boundary elements, (C) zoomed coarser mesh: complete mesh consists of 18,845 domain and 3633 boundary elements, (D) zoomed normal mesh: complete mesh consists of 29,514 domain and 4812 boundary elements, (E) zoomed finer mesh: complete mesh consists of 56,358 domain and 7154 boundary elements, (F) zoomed extremely fine mesh: complete mesh consists of 81,100 domain and 8470 boundary elements.

reveal another important result that as the nanofluid moves in the blood vessel and then from blood vessel to tumor interstitium, the peak values of velocity magnitude are shifting lowest values indicating the decrease of velocity during its flow. The velocity variation along with vertical line segments L4, L5, and L6 is demonstrated in Fig. 8.5E. This result shows that the velocity in the blood vessel parallel to the epithelial cell spacing is lower than the velocity in the blood vessel at the left edges of the epithelial cells. The velocity of the nanofluid shows a tendency to escape through the epithelial cell spacing.

In the second phase of our simulations, we have simulated the time-dependent concentration of the nanofluid from blood vessel to tumor interstitium at time $t = 0.00, 0.01, 0.05, 0.10, 0.15, 0.20$ s as shown in Fig. 8.6A, B, C, D, and E, respectively. For the solution of concentration in the tumor, the number of degrees of freedom solved was 68,016 (plus 11,033 internal DOFs) and solution time was $t = 229$ s (3 min, 49 s). The mass concentration at the inlet can be calculated following the expression $\gamma_c = \phi \times \rho_{nf} = 2086.94$ kg/m$^3 \approx 11{,}743.7$ mol/m$^3 \approx 11.7$

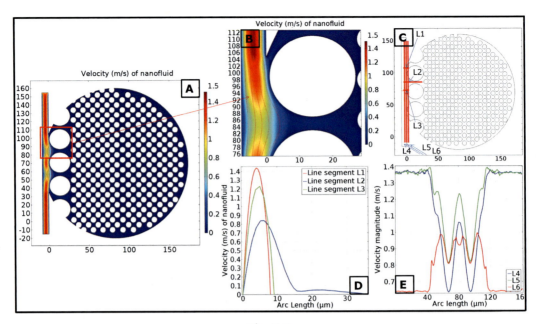

Fig. 8.5

Simulating steady-state velocity of the nanofluid: (A) surface plot of velocity distribution, (B) zoomed plot of (A), (C) visual clue of line segments, (D) behavior of nanofluid velocity for the horizontal line segments, and (E) behavior of nanofluid velocity for the vertical line segments.

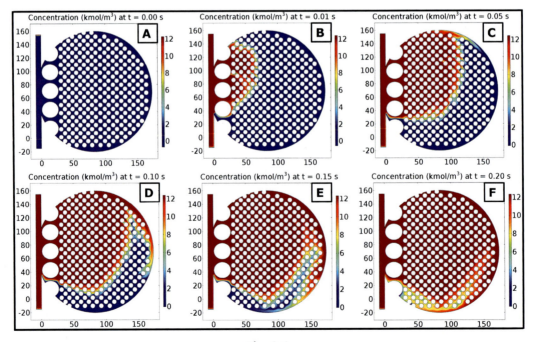

Fig. 8.6

Simulation of the nanofluid concentration: (A) the concentration of nanofluid at time $t = 0.00$ s, (B) the concentration of nanofluid at time $t = 0.01$ s, (C) the concentration of nanofluid at time $t = 0.05$ s, (D) the concentration of nanofluid at time $t = 0.10$ s, (E) the concentration of nanofluid at time $t = 0.15$ s, and (F) the concentration of nanofluid at time $t = 0.20$ s.

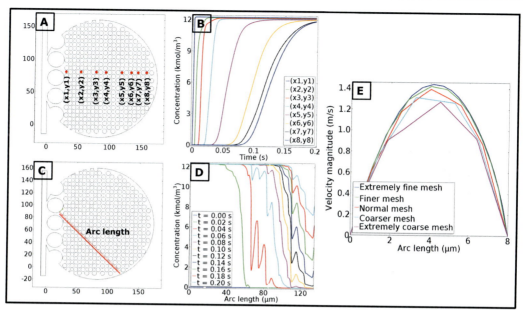

Fig. 8.7

Simulations of quantitative behavior of concentration: (A) visual clue of selected points in the tumor interstitium, (B) concentration versus time profiles in the tumor interstitium, (C) visual clue of the line segment, (D) concentration versus arc length curves along the selected line segment, and (E) mesh-dependent analysis of the nanofluid flow in the blood vessel.

kmol/m^3. The concentration of nanofluid is the maximum at the start of the process and the nanofluid moves slowly through the tumor interstitium. It is attenuated with time until the whole nanofluid is distributed throughout the tumor interstitium.

To investigate the concentration of the nanofluid quantitatively in the tumor interstitium, we have selected points $(x_i, y_j, i=j)$: $i, j = 1, 2, 3, 4, 5, 6, 7, 8$ as shown in Fig. 8.7A and the corresponding concentration versus time curves at these points are shown in Fig. 8.7B. These curves show that the concentration is maximum at point (x_1, x_1) and is minimum at point (x_8, x_8). This result shows that concentration decreases inflowing from the epithelial cell spacing to the entire tumor region.

For the prediction of concentration versus arc length in the tumor interstitium, we have selected a line segment whose visual clue is shown in Fig. 8.7C. The corresponding concentrations versus arc length curves along this line segment are demonstrated in Fig. 8.7D. This result shows that initially, the concentration in the tumor region near the blood vessel is zero because the nanofluid flowing in the blood vessel has not yet reached there. But with time concentration starts to increase and it becomes maximum after maximum elapsed time. The broken graphs represent the presence of tumor cells while the nanofluid moves through the pores. Lastly, the mesh-dependent analysis for the velocity of the nanofluid in the blood vessel is demonstrated in

Table 8.3 Mesh-dependent analysis.

Mesh type	Maximum element size (μm)	Minimum element size (μm)	Solution time (s)	No of degrees of freedom solved
Extremely fine	2	0.027	28	204,048
Finer	4	0.18	22	158,889
Normal	6	0.54	16	115,677
Coarser	8	0.9	10	64,839
Extremely coarse	10	1.26	05	35,283

Table 8.3 and Fig. 8.7E. As the mesh changes from coarser to finer mesh mode, the peak values of the velocity versus arc length curves are shifted to higher values. Extremely fine mesh mode produces more effective results than the remaining mesh modes.

Lastly, after the diffusion of nanofluid in the tumor, we have switched on the applied magnetic field, the MNPs start to oscillate and dissipate heat due to Neel and Brownian relaxational effects. The induced heat raised the temperature of the tumor. After 60 min of heating, the temperature elevation in the tumor is demonstrated in Fig. 8.8A. The maximum temperature is raised to 45°C from the body's normal temperature. For quantitative analysis of the temperature distribution, we have selected five points inside the tumor whose visual clue is also shown in the same diagram. The corresponding temperature versus time profiles at these selected points are

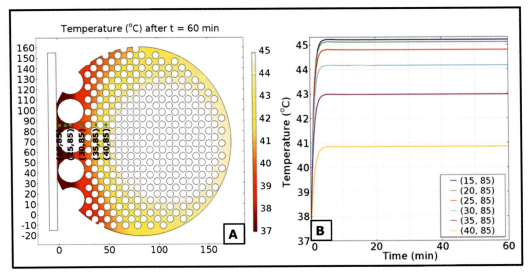

Fig. 8.8
Simulations of the temperature distribution in the tumor tissue, (A) 2D surface plot of temperature with selected points and (B) temperature versus time profiles at selected points.

shown in Fig. 8.8B. The results show that at the tumor center, the maximum temperature is obtained but as we move from the center toward the outside, the temperature starts to decrease and becomes minimum at the external edge of the tumor. This temperature is sufficient to kill the tumor cells under heat stress or cytotoxic effect.

8.4 Conclusions

The EPR effect and the nanofluid diffusion in the tumor to investigate their behaviors quantitatively for preheat generation planning has been simulated in hyperthermia treatment of cancer. The nanofluid velocity of moving fluid through the blood vessel is maximum at the center of the vessel and minimum near the outer walls of the vessel. The velocity of nanofluid at the inlet is larger as compared to the velocity at any other point in the blood vessel. While moving through the blood vessel, the velocity in the regions parallel to the epithelial cell spacing is maximum and minimum near in the regions parallel to the edges of the epithelial cells. The concentration of the nanofluid is the maximum near the blood vessel and it decreases as the nanofluid moves through the tumor interstitium. Both, the velocity, and concentration of nanofluid from blood vessels to tumor interstitium decrease with time. The mesh-dependent solution for the velocity in the blood vessel reveals that the extremely fine mesh mode produces the best solutions. This work will aid to control the accurate diffusion of nanofluid in porous tumors to produce effective and uniform heating in hyperthermia treatment of cancer.

References

[1] Wang M, Thanou M. Targeting nanoparticles to cancer. Pharmacol Res 2010;62:90–9.
[2] Allard E, Passirani C, Benoit J-P. Convection-enhanced delivery of nanocarriers for the treatment of brain tumors. Biomaterials 2009;30:2302–18.
[3] McGuire S, Zaharoff D, Yuan F. Nonlinear dependence of hydraulic conductivity on tissue deformation during intratumoral infusion. Ann Biomed Eng 2006;34:1173–81.
[4] Matsuki H, Yanada T, Sato T, Murakami K, Minakawa S. Temperature-sensitive amorphous magnetic flakes for intratissue hyperthermia. Mater Sci Eng A 1994;181:1366–8.
[5] Hilger I, Hergt R, Kaiser WA. Towards breast cancer treatment by magnetic heating. J Magn Magn Mater 2005;293:314–9.
[6] Salloum M, Ma R, Zhu L. Enhancement in treatment planning for magnetic nanoparticle hyperthermia: optimization of the heat absorption pattern. Int J Hyperth 2009;25:309–21.
[7] Iyer AK, Khaled G, Fang J, Maeda H. Exploiting the enhanced permeability and retention effect for tumor targeting. Drug Discov Today 2006;11:812–8.
[8] Dreher MR, Liu W, Michelich CR, Dewhirst MW, Yuan F, Chilkoti A. Tumor vascular permeability, accumulation, and penetration of macromolecular drug carriers. J Natl Cancer Inst 2006;98:335–44.
[9] de Lange DC, Engesæter BØ, Haug I, Ormberg I, Halgunset J, Brekken C. Uptake of IgG in osteosarcoma correlates inversely with interstitial fluid pressure, but not with interstitial constituents. Br J Cancer 2001;85:1968.
[10] Cho K, Wang X, Nie S, Shin DM. Therapeutic nanoparticles for drug delivery in cancer. Clin Cancer Res 2008;14:1310–6.
[11] Wei Y. Synthesis of Fe_3O_4 nanoparticles and their magnetic properties. arXiv 2020. preprint arXiv:200106583.

[12] Lim J, Yeap SP, Che HX, Low SC. Characterization of magnetic nanoparticle by dynamic light scattering. Nanoscale Res Lett 2013;8:381.

[13] Al-Waeli AH, Chaichan MT, Kazem HA, Sopian K, Safaei J. Numerical study on the effect of operating nanofluids of photovoltaic thermal system (PV/T) on the convective heat transfer. Case Stud Thermal Eng 2018;12:405–13.

[14] Javidi M, Heydari M, Karimi A, Haghpanahi M, Navidbakhsh M, Razmkon A. Evaluation of the effects of injection velocity and different gel concentrations on nanoparticles in hyperthermia therapy. J Biomed Phys Eng 2014;4:151.

[15] Hasgall P. ITIS database for thermal and electromagnetic parameters of biological tissues, version 2.2; July 11, 2012.

[16] Pennes HH. Analysis of tissue and arterial blood temperatures in the resting human forearm. J Appl Physiol 1948;1:93–122.

[17] Rosensweig RE. Heating magnetic fluid with alternating magnetic field. J Magn Magn Mater 2002;252:370–4.

[18] Miaskowski A, Sawicki B. Magnetic fluid hyperthermia modeling based on phantom measurements and realistic breast model. IEEE Trans Biomed Eng 2013;60:1806–13.

# CHAPTER 9

Simulating the nanoflow around Happel's sphere in the porous tumor carrying the cell-model structure

In drug delivery studies, selection of unit structural cells of porous tissue is the main challenge owing to the presence of an extracellular matrix. The porous tissue structures are considered to be a matrix of spherical cells [1]. Collagen tries to hinder diffusion in molecules, generally in large sizes. Due to limited research on the topic, it is ambiguous as to what limit the extracellular matrix impacts the convective transport of fluid. We generally exclude the collagen fibers in the unit cell and for an ideal case, we also neglect the extracellular matrix and take the HS as unit structural cells for tumor tissue [2]. HS in cell models [3] is the structural unit cells of granular porous media. The cell is represented by a solid spherical body with diameter a_c surrounded by a fluid layer with thickness, $\gamma = (a_c/2)((1-\varepsilon)^{-1/3} - 1)$ [4].

Among the limited studies, the mentionable work related to HS includes the first analytical treatment of the slow motion of fluid relative to HS by Happel [3]. This study was based on general assumptions and boundary conditions. A closed-form solution was obtained which satisfied the Navier-Stokes equation neglecting inertia terms. His theoretical formulation agreed well with the experimental data of Carman-Kozeny. Later, Rajagopal and Tien [5] developed analytical models of particle deposition and trajectory analysis in deep bed filter taking into consideration HS in the cell model. Lecoanet and Wiesner [6] studied velocity effects on fullerene and oxide MNPs. They considered porous media and adopted a theoretical framework based on the HS cell model. Levine [7] predicted electrophoresis and electro-osmosis where the electrophoretic velocity of a swarm of the solid sphere was adopted from Happel's sphere.

Besides the above prominent approaches toward HS, no author has yet treated the HS from the computational modeling approach. We have conducted an in silico study of the nanofluid flow of iron oxide MNPs in the porous tumors. We will develop numerical FEM models for simulations of velocity and concentration in the porous tumors around HS. To the author's best knowledge, this is the first numerical study where nanoflow is simulated to investigate its behavior in a porous matrix considering HS in the cell model. We will simulate the nanoflow in porous tumors and investigate how it behaves near a structural unit of porous tumor, which is assumed to be HS. We will simulate nanoflow through the cubical and hexagonal packed structure of porous tumor matrix. We will also investigate the mesh-dependent analysis of the velocity of the nanofluid.

9.1 Physical properties of nanofluids

In the present study, we will take Fe_3O_4 MNPs of size 15nm and the base fluid deionized water (DIW) with densities $\rho_p = 3890 kg/m^3$ and $\rho_{bf} = 997.1 kg/m^3$, respectively [8]. The properties of nanofluids have been calculated in the supplementary material: Appendix B, which we will use in simulations.

9.2 Mathematical modeling formulation of the problem

9.2.1 Nanofluid flow in the porous tumor

Nanofluid flow in the porous tumor is modeled through the Navier-Stokes equation (4.1) coupled with the continuity equation, where ρ_{nf} is the density of the nanofluid and η is the dynamic viscosity of the nanofluid. The IC includes both the velocity and pressure being zero in the tumor as demonstrated below:

$$\boldsymbol{u} = 0, \boldsymbol{p} = 0 \tag{9.1}$$

The BC include that the inlet is

$$\boldsymbol{u} = -U_0 n \tag{9.2}$$

where U_0 is the inflow velocity of the nanofluid in the blood vessel that can be calculated using the expression

$$U_0 = Q/A \tag{9.3}$$

where Q is the flow rate of the nanofluid at the inlet which we are taking $3\mu L/min$ and A is the area of the cross section for the rectangle (Domain 1), which is calculated to be $5.03 \times 10^{-11} m^2$ with the radius 25μm. The inflow velocity at the inlet becomes $9.95 \times 10^{-1} m/s$ and the outlet is defined as

$$-p\boldsymbol{I} + \eta\left(\nabla \boldsymbol{u} + (\nabla \boldsymbol{u})^T\right)n = -\widehat{p}_0 n, \quad \widehat{p}_0 \leq p_0 \tag{9.4}$$

9.2.2 Nanofluid diffusion in the tumor interstitium

Transport of the nanofluid in the porous tumor is modeled through the convection-diffusion equation (4.4). We are considering only the convection-enhanced diffusion of the nanofluid and neglecting the microscale interactions of the nanofluid with the tumor matrix while flowing through it. The D^k is the diffusion coefficient that can be calculated by using the Stokes-Einstein equation (4.5), where $k_B = 1.38 \times 10^{-23}$ J/K is the Boltzmann constant, $T = 310.15$K is the absolute temperature, $\eta_{nf} = 0.01722$ Pas is the viscosity of nanofluid, and $r_p = 7.5$ nm is the radius of a nanoparticle. Using these values, D_0 is calculated to be 5.94×10^{-11} m²/s. L is the factor responsible for the hydrodynamic and steric reduction of the diffusion coefficient in the pore, $F > 1$ is the shape factor that accounts for hindrance in the pores, and $\tau(\varepsilon)$ is tortuosity due to increased diffusion path length. The values of D^k become 4.95×10^{-11} m²/s where the values of L, F, and τ are taken 1, 2, and 0.6 [9], respectively. The IC includes zero initial concentration in all domains:

$$c^k = 0 \qquad (9.5)$$

and BC includes no flux at the outer boundary of the tissue

$$-n \cdot N^k = 0 \qquad (9.6)$$

9.3 Results

From the model wizard, the physics for the nanofluid flow is selected as *laminar flow* from the *single-phase flow* node which was selected from the *fluid-flow* node. For nanofluid diffusion around the Happel's sphere, the physics of the *convection-diffusion equation* was selected from the *transport of diluted species (chds)* node that was selected from the *chemical species transport* node. The studies for *laminar flow* and *convection-diffusion equation* were selected as stationary and time-dependent, respectively. For the geometry of the problem, Happel's sphere was constructed with diameter ∼20 μm surrounded by a fluid layer with thickness ∼1 μm enclosed in a rectangle of width ∼50μm, and length ∼70μm, as shown in Fig. 9.1. We are taking this rectangle as a porous tumor matrix.

The ICs and BCs were inserted as defined in the respective sections of each physics. Inlet velocity was inserted as $U_0 = 9.95 \times 10^{-1}$ m/s and outlet pressure is taken as $p = 0$ Pa. For the convection-diffusion equation, the mass concentration at the inlet was inserted to be $\gamma_c = \phi \times \rho_{nf} = 2086.94$ kg/m³ $\approx 11{,}743.7$ mol/m³ ≈ 11.7 kmol/m³ and the initial value of the concentration was taken as $c = 0$ mol/m³. The material's Domain 1 was taken as the liver and Domain 2 was taken as liquid/water. After adding physics, corresponding studies, materials, ICs, and BCs, the mesh was generated in extremely fine mesh mode as shown in Fig. 9.2 where the details about the generated mesh are narrated in the caption.

The model (4.1) was simulated for the velocity of nanofluid flow around HS as demonstrated in Fig. 9.3. The velocity is maximum below and at the upper side of HS and minimum near walls and moderates at the inlet and outlet of the HS.

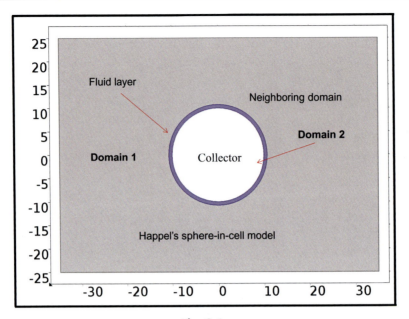

Fig. 9.1
HS in porous tumor matrix where the collector is surrounded by a fluid layer.

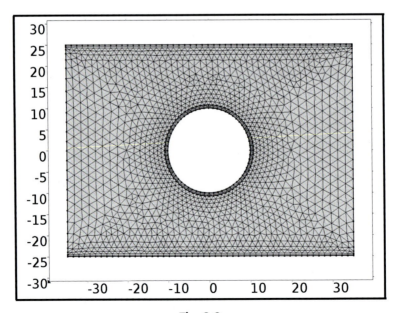

Fig. 9.2
Mesh generation of the problem in an extremely fine mesh mode. The complete mesh consists of 29,890 elements, 960 boundary elements, maximum element size is 0.65μm, minimum element size is 0.0075μm, maximum element growth is 1.08, curvature factor is 0.25, and the resolution of the narrow region is 1.

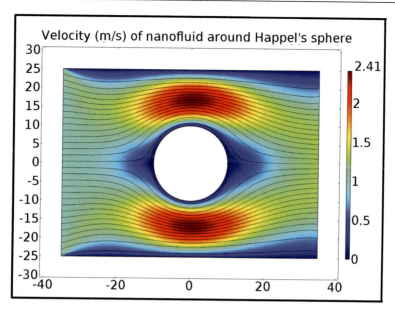

Fig. 9.3
Velocity distribution of the nanofluid around Happel's sphere with streamlines.

To investigate the behavior of the nanoflow surrounding the HS quantitatively, we have selected two-line segments Cut Line 2D1 and Cut Line 2D2 along the width and length of the rectangle whose visual clues are shown in Fig. 9.4A. The behavior of the velocity along Cut Line 2D1 is demonstrated in Fig. 9.4B. The velocity is maximum at the upper and lower regions of the HS whereas velocity is minimum at the front boundary of the HS where nanofluid hits the HS from the left side. The nanofluid shows a tendency to escape the regions around HS. The velocity along Cut Line 2D2 is shown in Fig. 9.4C. The result shows that the velocity is maximum at the inlet and decreases as the nanofluid moves toward the HS. and becomes minimum on hitting the boundary and after, escaping around the sphere, the velocity again starts to increase and becomes maximum at the outlet.

Next, we performed a mesh-dependent analysis for the velocity of nanofluid. We have computationally solved model (4.1) for velocity by generating meshes in extremely fine, finer, fine, coarser, and extremely coarser mesh modes. The velocity distribution for each of the mesh mode is simulated along with the line segment Cut Line 2D3 as demonstrated in Fig. 9.5, where the visual clue of the Cut Line 2D3 is shown in the left upper corner of Fig. 9.5. The result reveals that as the mesh becomes more and finer, the solution curve shifts to a higher position, and velocity increases through the small amount. The details of the mesh modes are shown in Table 9.1.

Next, we have simulated the diffusion model (4.4) for the concentration of the nanofluid around HS. The concentration at selected times $t=0, 1, 3, 5, 10, 15, 20, 25\,s$ is demonstrated in

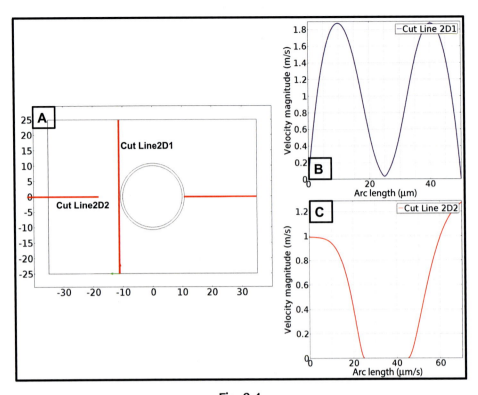

Fig. 9.4
Quantitative analysis of the velocity of nanofluid around Happel's sphere: (A) visual clues of line segments: Cut Line 2D1 and Cut Line 2D2, (B) velocity of nanofluid along Cut Line 2D1, and (C) velocity of nanofluid along with Cut Line 2D2.

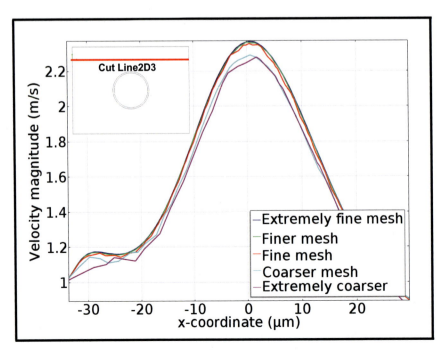

Fig. 9.5
Mesh-dependent analysis of the velocity of nanofluid in the porous tumors.

Table 9.1 Quantitative analysis of the mesh-dependent velocity of the nanofluid.

Mesh	Vortex elements	Boundary element	Total elements	Minimum element quality
Extremely fine	12	960	29,870	0.7349
Finer	12	916	19,438	0.8008
Fine	12	484	7140	0.7473
Coarser	12	276	2912	0.7071
Extremely coarser	12	260	2022	0.7270

Figs. 9.6 and 9.7. From both the figures, it is evident that as the time elapses, the concentration moves from the inlet to the outlet crossing the HS and escaping from the below and upper regions of the HS. To investigate the concentration quantitatively, we have selected points x_1, x_2, x_3, x_4, x_5, x_6, and x_7 in the tumor matrix whose visual clue is shown in Fig. 9.8A. The concentration versus time plots at these selected points is shown in Fig. 9.8B. The concentration at point x_1 is maximum as compared to the concentration at the point x_7 where the concentration

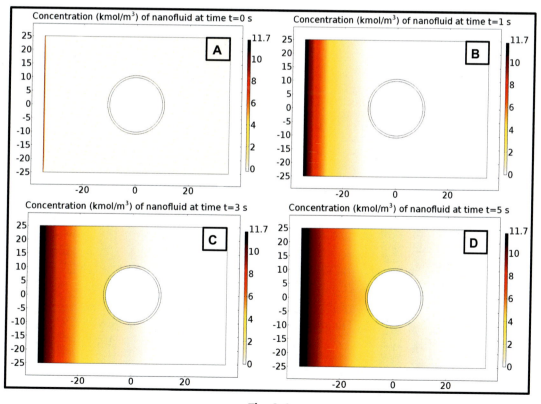

Fig. 9.6

Simulation of concentration of the nanofluid: (A) concentration at $t=0$ s, (B) concentration at $t=1$ s, (C) concentration at $t=3$ s, and (D) concentration at $t=5$ s.

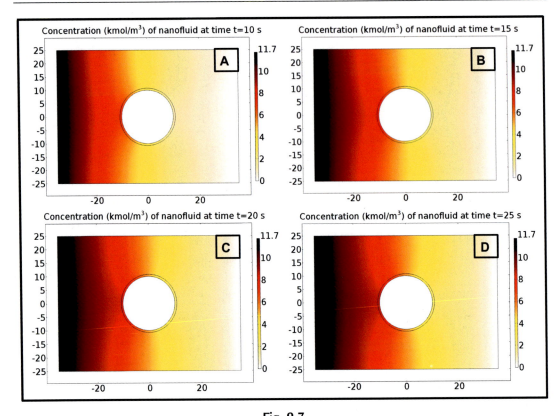

Fig. 9.7
Simulation of concentration of the nanofluid: (A) concentration at $t=10\,s$, (B) concentration at $t=15\,s$, (C) concentration at $t=20\,s$, and (D) concentration at $t=25\,s$.

is minimum. At the remaining points, the concentration decreases from the maximum concentration to the minimum concentration. The result reveals that the concentration decreases as the nanofluid moves from the inlet to the HS. To investigate the concentration of nanofluid after crossing the HS, we have selected points x_8, x_9, x_{10}, x_{11}, x_{12}, x_{13}, and x_{14} in the tumor matrix whose visual clue is shown in Fig. 9.8A. The concentration versus time plots at these selected points are shown in Fig. 9.8C. The concentration at point x_8 is maximum as compared to the concentration at point x_{14} where the concentration is minimum. At the remaining points, the concentration decreases from the maximum concentration to the minimum concentration. The result reveals that the concentration decreases when the nanofluid moves from HS to the outlet.

The nanofluid flow is simulated through the cubical and hexagonal arrangement of the HS as shown in Fig. 9.9A and B, respectively. The simulation shows different behaviors of the nanofluid in both structures. The nanofluid flow through the cubical arrangement of the porous structure is smoother than the hexagonal package. In the hexagonal package, the nanofluid

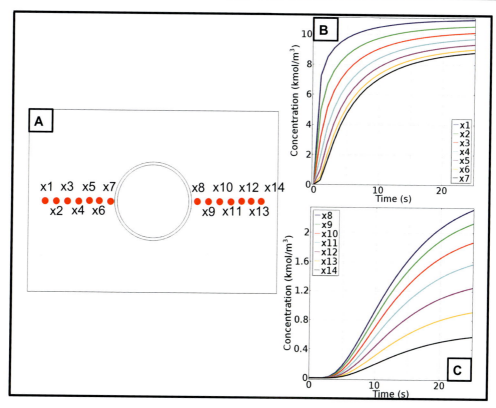

Fig. 9.8
Simulation of the concentration of the nanofluid quantitatively: (A) visual clue of the selected points, (B) concentration versus time plots at the selected points from inlet to the HS, and (C) concentration versus time plots at the selected points from HS to outlet.

faces more deviation than other approaches and it affects the diffusion of the nanofluid in the porous tissue. Moreover, the velocity of the nanoflow is maximum between voids of the HS as compared to the remaining space.

For investigating the behavior of the nanofluid through these structures quantitatively, we have selected two-line segments Cut Line 2D4 and Cut Line 2D5 on each structure whose visual clue is shown in Fig. 9.10A and C, respectively. The velocity of the nanofluid through cubical structure along this line segment Fig. 9.10A is demonstrated in Fig. 9.10B. The simulation result shows that the velocity through the voids is maximum and is minimum in spacing between two adjacent spheres in the normal direction to the flow. Moreover, velocity curves are periodic in the cubical structure. The velocity of the nanofluid through a hexagonal structure along the line segment Cut Line 2D5 is simulated in Fig. 9.10D. Again, the velocity through the voids is maximum. Higher velocity peaks are neither equally spaced nor with equal heights.

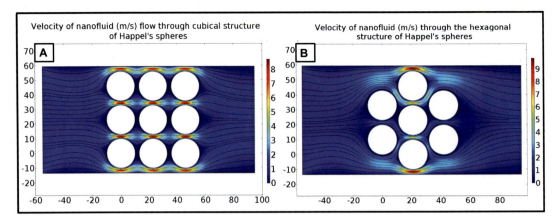

Fig. 9.9

Simulation of the concentration of the nanofluid: (A) through cubical structure and (B) through hexagonal structure.

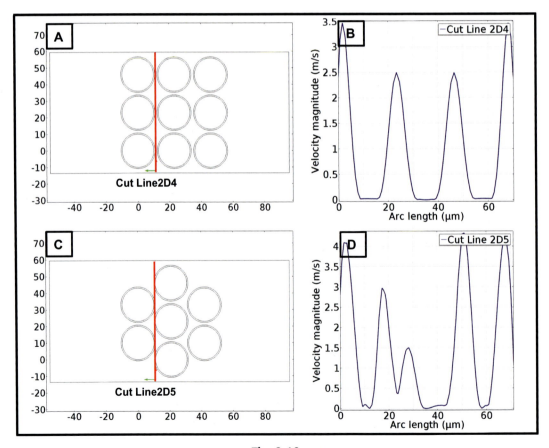

Fig. 9.10

Quantitative prediction of nanofluid velocity: (A) visual clue of the line segment, cut line 2D4 in cubical structure, (B) velocity versus arc length along with the Cut Line 2D4, (C) visual clue of line segment, Cut Line 2D5 in the hexagonal structure, and (D) velocity versus arc length along the Cut Line 2D5.

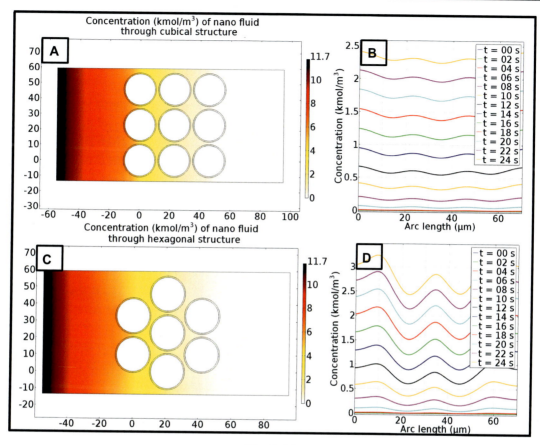

Fig. 9.11
Simulation of the concentration of the nanofluid: (A) through cubical structure, (B) concentration versus arc length at selected times, (C) through hexagonal structure, and (D) concentration versus arc length at selected times.

Moreover, the distribution of velocity is nonperiodic. The velocity attained in the hexagonal structure is also higher than the velocity magnitude attained in the cubical structure. Thus, the nanofluid moves fast in the hexagonal structure of porous tissue.

The simulation of the concentration of nanofluid in the cubical structure is shown in Fig. 9.11A and the quantitative behavior of concentration versus arc length at selected times is shown in Fig. 9.11B. The result shows that the concentration curves are smoother with small deviations. The simulation of concentration of nanofluid in the hexagonal structure is shown in Fig. 9.11C and the quantitative behavior of concentration versus arc length at selected times is shown in Fig. 9.11D. The result shows that the concentration curves are more deviated as compared to the previous case. Thus, the simulation results show that the nanofluid is turbulent in hexagonal structure and laminar in the cubical structure.

9.4 Conclusions

The nanofluid around HS in the cell model in cubical and hexagonal packaging is simulated and analyzed quantitatively. The velocity of the nanoflow is maximum below and the upper region of the sphere and concentration decreases from inlet to the HS and then from HS to the outlet. The nanofluid moves through the hexagonal structure with more turbulent flow and with fast speed as compared with the cubical structure. The velocity of the nanofluid in a cubical structure follows some periodicity but in the hexagonal structure, no such periodicity was observed. Nanoflow in a hexagonal structure is more deviated than the cubical structure. The concentration is also smoother in cubical structure as compared to the hexagonal package. An extremely fine mesh produces better numerical solutions than other mesh modes. One of the recommendations from the current research is that for hexagonal tumor structure, magnetic fluid hyperthermia will be more effective than with cubical structure. The finer the mesh better will be the solution with a minor addition to the velocity. The velocity of the nanofluid through voids is a maximum and the flow-through of the cubical structure is smoother than the hexagonal structure. The flow is more turbulent and faster in the porous hexagonal structure. This research will aid hyperthermia treatment protocols for cancer patients in clinical applications.

References

[1] Chen Z-J, Broaddus WC, Viswanathan RR, Raghavan R, Gillies GT. Intraparenchymal drug delivery via positive-pressure infusion: experimental and modeling studies of poroelasticity in brain phantom gels. IEEE Trans Biomed Eng 2002;49:85–96.
[2] Netti PA, Baxter LT, Boucher Y, Skalak R, Jain RK. Macro-and microscopic fluid transport in living tissues: application to solid tumors. AIChE J 1997;43:818–34.
[3] Happel J. Viscous flow in multiparticle systems: slow motion of fluids relative to beds of spherical particles. AIChE J 1958;4:197–201.
[4] Nelson KE, Ginn TR. Colloid filtration theory and the Happel sphere-in-cell model revisited with direct numerical simulation of colloids. Langmuir 2005;21:2173–84.
[5] Rajagopalan R, Tien C. Trajectory analysis of deep-bed filtration with the sphere-in-cell porous media model. AIChE J 1976;22:523–33.
[6] Lecoanet HF, Wiesner MR. Velocity effects on fullerene and oxide nanoparticle deposition in porous media. Environ Sci Technol 2004;38:4377–82.
[7] Levine S, Neale GH. The prediction of electrokinetic phenomena within multiparticle systems. I. Electrophoresis and electroosmosis. J Colloid Interface Sci 1974;47:520–9.
[8] Al-Waeli AH, Chaichan MT, Kazem HA, Sopian K, Safaei J. Numerical study on the effect of operating nanofluids of photovoltaic thermal system (PV/T) on the convective heat transfer. Case Stud Therm Eng 2018;12:405–13.
[9] Bear J. Dynamics of fluids in porous media. Courier Corporation; 2013.

CHAPTER 10

Computational analysis of the reacting nanofluid in the porous tumor

Chemical reactions, for instance, radioactive decay, exothermic reactions, or endothermic reactions, affect fluid transport in a porous medium. These reactions indicate, the time rate of change of concentration of fluid flow per unit volume of porous media [1–7]. Historically, the nanofluid flow of diluted species in the porous tumor was originally studied by Buongiorno [8]. Notable literature regarding the modeling of transport of macroparticles and microparticles in tumors includes the work by Banerjee et al. [9], who used a numerical modeling approach to simulate the antibody delivery to tumors. In the study [10], Graff and Wittrup simulated the antibody delivery to tumor spheroids using FEM models. In the study [11], Kwok et al. assumed structural uniformity while modeling tumor spheroids. In work [12], Wenning and Murphy assumed heterogeneous distribution of binding sites. The model in the study [10] was further extended by Goodman et al. [13] considering the nonuniformity of the spheroid in the radial direction and internalization of particles. The transport model [10] was also extended by Waite and Roth [14] considering binding and transport of PAMAM-RGD in a tumor spheroid model.

10.1 Properties of nanofluid

In this present study we will use Fe_3O_4 MNPs of size 15 nm and base fluid de-ionized water (DIW) with densities $\rho_p = 3890 \text{ kg/m}^3$ and $\rho_{bf} = 997.1 \text{ kg/m}^3$, respectively [15]. The properties of nanofluids have been calculated in Section 11.2.1, which we will use in simulations.

10.2 Mathematical modeling formulation of the problem

Our model of interest *reacting flow in porous media* contains three models: (1) Navier-Stokes equation, (2) diffusion-convection model, and (3) Brinkman model associated with Bruggeman effective transport parameter. The Navier-Stokes equation will simulate the velocity of the laminar flow of nanofluid through the tumor interstitium. The diffusion-convection model will simulate the nanofluid diffusion associated with reaction rates. The Brinkman model [16] will be used to simulate the velocity of nanoflow in porous tumor interstitium. This model contains a second-order term that allows the use of no-slip boundary conditions. Our complete coupled model is described as

$$\left.\begin{array}{l} \rho_{nf}(u \cdot \nabla)u = \nabla \cdot \left(-pI + \eta\left(\nabla u + (\nabla u)^T\right)\right) + F \\ \rho_{nf}(\nabla \cdot u) = 0 \end{array}\right\} \text{Navier} - \text{Stokes} - \text{equations}$$

$$\nabla \cdot \left(-D_i \nabla c_i - z_i u_{m,j} F c_i + \nabla v + u \cdot \nabla c_i\right) = R_i \} \text{Diffusion} - \text{convection} - \text{chemical} \\ -\text{reaction} - \text{kinetics}$$

$$\left.\begin{array}{l} N_i = -D_{i,\mathit{eff}} \nabla c_i + u c_i \\ D_{i,\mathit{eff}} = f_{\mathit{eff}} D_i, f_{\mathit{eff}} = \varepsilon_p^{3/2} \end{array}\right\} \text{Bruggeman} - \text{effective} - \text{transport} - \text{parameter}$$

$$\left.\begin{array}{l} \dfrac{\rho_{nf}}{\varepsilon_p}\left((u \cdot \nabla)\dfrac{u}{\varepsilon_p}\right) = \nabla \cdot \left[-pI + \dfrac{\eta}{\varepsilon_p}\left(\nabla u + (\nabla u)^T\right) - \dfrac{2\eta}{3\varepsilon_p}(\nabla \cdot u)I\right] \\ -\left(\eta K^{-1} + \beta_F |u| + \dfrac{Q_{br}}{\varepsilon_p^2}\right)u + F \\ \rho_{nf}(\nabla \cdot u) = Q_{br} \end{array}\right\} \text{Brinkman} - \text{equation}$$

(10.1)

In the above model, η represents the viscosity of the nanofluid (Pa s), ρ_{nf} is the density of nanofluid (kg/m^3), u the velocity of nanofluid (m/s), ε_p the porosity (dimensionless), K the permeability (m^2), F the external force (zero here), c_i the concentration (mol/m^3), R_i the reaction rate for the species i [mol/(m^3 s)], D_i the diffusion coefficient (m^2/s), Q_{br} the optional source term that accounts for mass deposit and mass creation within the domains (kg/(m^3 s)), and p the pressure (Pa). The terms $-z_i u_{m,j} F c_i + \nabla v$ are applicable only when migration in the electric field is also considered. Therefore, for the current study, we neglect these terms. The ICs include the concentration, velocity field, and pressure being zero in all domains as given below

$$c_1 = 0, \quad c_2 = 0, \quad c_3 = 0, \quad u = (0, 0, 0), \quad p = 0 \qquad (10.2)$$

and the BCs associated with this model are expressed below. The no flux condition is

$$-n \cdot N_i = 0 \qquad (10.3)$$

The wall is expressed as

$$u = 0 \qquad (10.4)$$

The reactions rates are formulated as

$$R_1 = -k c_1 c_2, \quad R_2 = -k c_1 c_2, \quad R_3 = k c_1 c_2 \qquad (10.5)$$

All in units of mol/(m^3 s). The reaction k is defined as

$$k = A e^{-\left(\frac{E_a}{R_u T}\right)} \qquad (10.6)$$

where $A = 1 \times 10^6$ m^3(s mol), $E = 30 \times 10^3$ J/mol, and $T = 310.15$ K. The inlet 1 is formulated as

$$u_1 = -U_{0,1}n_1 \tag{10.7}$$

where $U_{0,1} = 0.5 \times 10^{-3}$ m/s [17] is the velocity of blood species and inlet 2 is expressed as

$$u_2 = -U_{0,2}n_2 \tag{10.8}$$

where $U_{0,2} = 4.44 \times 10^{-12}$ m/s is the velocity of nanofluid that is calculated from the relation $Q = U_{0,2}A$ where the flow rate is taken to be 3 μL/min and A is the area of cross section of the needle. The outlet is expressed as

$$-p\mathbf{I} + \eta\left(\nabla u + (\nabla u)^T\right)n = -\widehat{p}_0 n$$
$$\widehat{p}_0 \leq p_0 \tag{10.9}$$

The symmetry 1 is defined as

$$u \cdot n = 0$$
$$k - (k \cdot n)n = 0, \quad k = \mu\left((\nabla u) + (\nabla u)^T\right)n \tag{10.10}$$

The inflow 1 is

$$c_1 = \gamma_b \tag{10.11}$$

and inflow 2 is

$$c_2 = \gamma_{nf} \tag{10.12}$$

where γ_b and γ_{nf} are mass concentrations and will be calculated later in Section 12.4. The outflow is

$$-n \cdot D_i \nabla c_i = 0 \tag{10.13}$$

Lastly, the symmetry 2 is defined as

$$-n \cdot N_i = 0 \tag{10.14}$$

10.3 Adding physics and geometry construction of the problem

From the model wizard, the 3D space dimension was selected. The physics was selected as reacting flow in porous media associated with stationary study for steady-state analysis. This physics carries the three models: (1) Navier-Stokes equation, (2) diffusion-convection model, and (3) Brinkman model. This physics is compatible with the model (10.1). The length units were in mm and angular units were in degrees. A cylinder of radius 4 mm and height 2 mm at position (0,0,0) and axis (1,0,0) was generated which acts as a porous-free space. The second cylinder of radius 6 mm and height 11 mm at position (2,0,0) and axis (1,0,0) was generated which acts as a porous tumor interstitium. The third cylinder of radius 4 mm and height 2 mm at position (13,0,0) and axis (1,0,0) was generated which acts as a porous free space. For constructing a needle, the fourth cylinder of radius 0.4mm and height 6mm at position (7.5,0,0) with axis type of z-axis was constructed. The fifth cylinder of radius 0.3mm and height 6mm at position (7.5,0,0) with axis type of z-axis was constructed. A block of width 12mm, depth 10 mm, and height 12mm with position (0,−10,−6) with axis type z-axis was generated. Compositions were used for all cylinders and block to generate the output geometry as shown in Fig. 10.1A with side view shown in Fig. 10.1B, and backside in Fig. 10.1C.

10.4 Adding initial condition, boundary conditions, and material

Our geometry consists of three domains, domain 2 serves as a porous tumor, and domain 1 and domain 3 act as porous-free space. For the transport properties, domains 1, 2, and 3 were selected as shown in Fig. 10.2A. The density of nanofluid was added 3006 kg/m³ and it was calculated from Eq. (4.15). The dynamic viscosity was added 0.01722 Pas and it was calculated from Eq. (4.18). The value of the diffusion coefficient was inserted as $D_i = 1.76 \times 10^{-12}$ m²/s and it was calculated from Eq. (4.5). No flux condition was applied on the boundaries 3–5, 7, 9, 10–16, 19, 20. Wall with the no-slip condition was applied to the same boundaries. The ICs were added from Eq. (10.2) in all three domains. For porous matrix properties, domain 2 was selected.

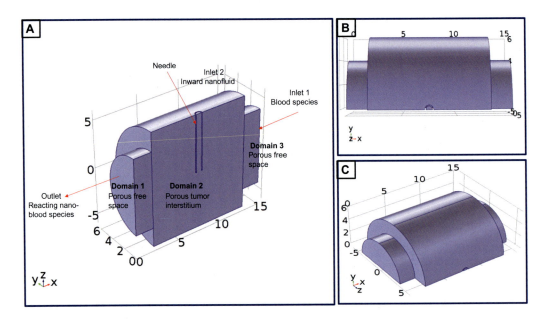

Fig. 10.1
Geometry of the problem: (A) geometry of porous tissue surrounded by porous free regions and injected needle in the tumor, (B) side view of the geometry with the needle at the bottom, and (C) arial view of the porous tumor interstitium.

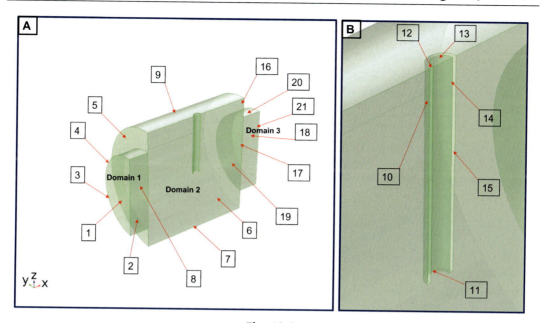

Fig. 10.2
Boundaries of the model: (A) boundaries of the three domains and (B) boundaries of the zoomed needle.

The porosity of tumor was added as $\epsilon_p=0.8$ [18] and permeability $K=1\times 10^{-17}\,\text{m}^2$ [18]. The effective mass transport parameter was selected as Bruggeman as defined in the model (10.1). The reactions for domain 2 were added as described in Eqs. (10.5) and (10.6). The velocity of blood species was added as inlet 1 at boundary 21 and the velocity of nanofluid was added as inlet 2 at boundary 13. The velocities of blood and nanofluid have been calculated in Eqs. (10.7) and (10.8), respectively. The pressure $p=0$Pa was added at the outlet at boundary 1. Symmetry was added at boundaries 2, 6, and 18. The mass concentration of the nanofluid 1901 mol/m³ was added as inflow 1 at the boundary 21, which was calculated as $\gamma_{nf}=\phi\times\rho_{nf}=0.6943\times 3006=2086.94$ kg/m³. But the molar mass of Fe_3O_4 MNPs is 159.687 g/mol = 0.159687 kg/mol and the molar mass of base fluid water is 18.02 g/mol = 0.01802 kg/mol. Therefore, molar mass of nanofluid is 177.71 g/mol = 0.1777 kg/mol. The mass concentration of nanofluid $\gamma_{nf}=2086.94/0.1777=11{,}743.74$ mol/m³. Similarly, the mass concentration of the blood species $\gamma_b=\phi\times\rho_{nf}=33\%\times 1025=388.25$ kg/m³ ≈ 388.25 mol/m³ was added as inflow 1 at the boundary 13, where the density of the blood species is 1025 kg/m³ and volume fraction is 30%–36% [19] with the average value of 33%. The outflow was added at boundary 1. Symmetry 2 was added at the boundaries 2, 6, and 18. Since oxygen is the prominent constituent of the tissue, we have added oxygen/water/liquid material for all domains 1, 2, and 3. For simplicity of the model, we ignore the microscale interactions of the blood species with porous matrix and between blood cells. Our focus is on the blood reacting with nanofluid coming from the needle and gives product at the outlet.

10.5 Mesh generation of the problem

After adding physics, studies, ICs, BCs, a mesh was generated in fine mesh mode as shown in Fig. 10.3A, zoom mesh of the needle in Fig. 10.3B, and zoom needle at the inlet 2 shown in Fig. 10.3C. The mesh details are given in the caption.

10.6 Results and discussions

After generating the mesh, the model (10.1) was solved and it resulted in the solution for velocity, pressure, and concentration of the nanofluid simultaneously. The simulation of velocity is demonstrated in Fig. 10.4A. The reacting flow is almost homogenous in the porous part of the tissue. The maximum velocity of the nanofluid is achieved by 50.1 mm/s. Along the line segments L1 and L2 in Fig. 10.4A, the velocity magnitude versus z-coordinate have been simulated quantitatively as shown in Fig. 10.4B. This result shows that the velocity at the inlet 1 is higher than the velocity at the outlet. The velocity decreases after passing through the porous medium. The velocity along the line segment L3 is simulated in Fig. 10.4C. The velocity is in a parabolic shape, maximum at the center and minimum near the walls.

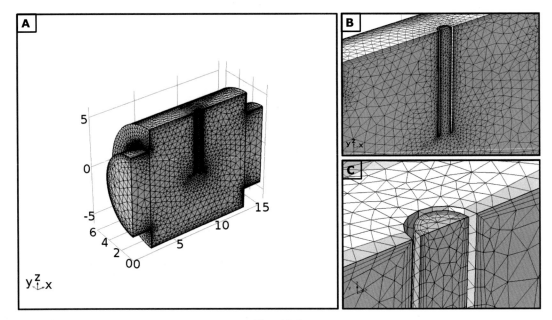

Fig. 10.3
Geometry of the problem: no. of elements: 172,386, vortex elements: 30, edge elements: 1140, boundary elements: 24,206, free meshing time: 7.72 s, minimum element quality: 0.1529, maximum element size: 1.2 mm, minimum elements size: 0.15, maximum element growth rate: 1.45, curvature factor: 0.5, and resolution of narrow regions 0.6.

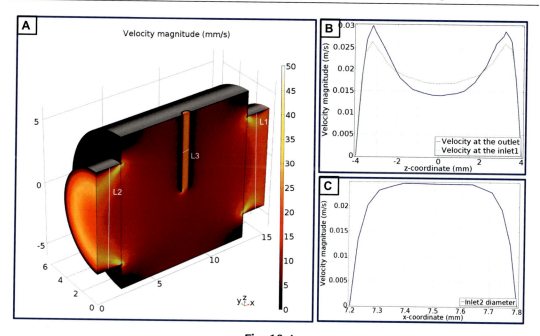

Fig. 10.4

Simulation of the velocity of nanofluid: (A) 3D velocity distribution, (B) velocity versus z-coordinate along with L1 and L2, and (C) velocity versus x-coordinate along with L3.

The pressure distribution of nanofluid in the tissue is shown in Fig. 10.5A and the line plot along the line segment L1 in Fig. 10.5A is plotted in Fig. 10.5B. These results show that pressure drops across the porous tissue. The pressure is maximum at the inlet 1 and minimum at the outlet.

The concentration c_1 of the nanofluid is simulated as demonstrated in Fig. 10.6A whose zoomed surface plot is shown in Fig. 10.6B and the isosurface plot is shown in Fig. 10.6C. These results show that concentration decreases rapidly with the distance from the point of injection. Moreover, the maximum concentration obtained is $11.8\,kmol/m^3$.

The slice plot for the concentration c_1 is demonstrated in Fig. 10.7A. To analyze the results quantitatively, we have drawn line segments L1, L2, L3, L4, and L5 in Fig. 10.7A, and the corresponding concentration line graphs along these line segments are shown in Fig. 10.7B. The peak values of the concentration decrease with increase in the distance from the injecting position.

The concentration of blood species c_2 is simulated in Fig. 10.8A. The reaction is not uniformly distributed in the porous medium and has a maximum close to the radial position of the injecting point. The line plots along with the selected line segments L1, L2, L3, L4, and L5 in Fig. 10.8A show that a low concentration is attained near the injecting point.

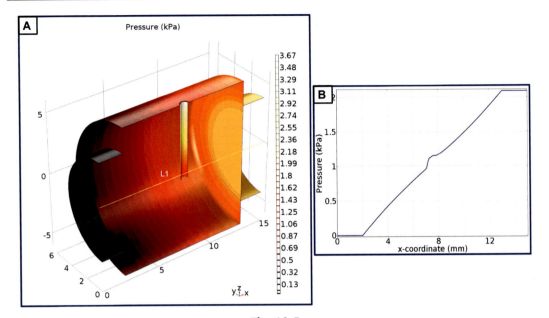

Fig. 10.5
Pressure distribution in the tissue: (A) 3D pressure distribution and (B) pressure versus *x*-coordinate along L1.

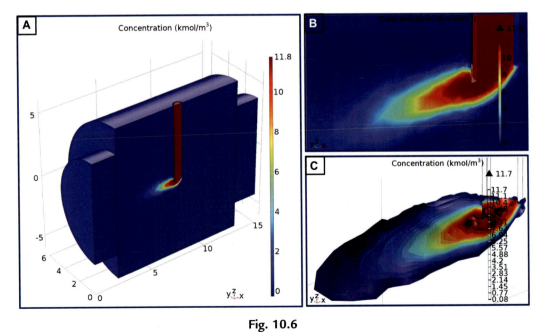

Fig. 10.6
Simulation of nanofluid species: (A) 3D distribution of concentration, (B) zoomed plot of concentration, and (C) zoomed isosurface plot.

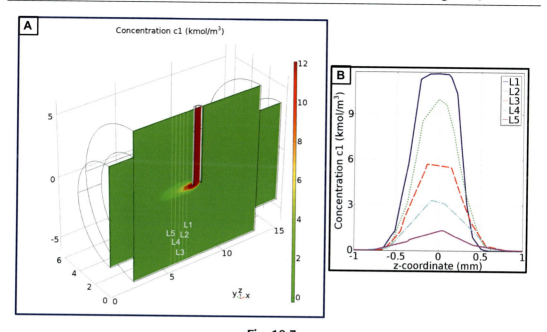

Fig. 10.7
Concentration of nanofluid species: (A) slice plot of concentration c_1 with the visual clue of the line segments and (B) line plots of concentration versus z-coordinate at selected line segments.

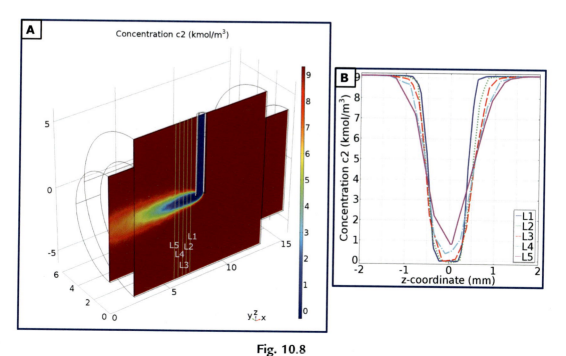

Fig. 10.8
Simulation of blood species: (A) slice plot of concentration c_2 with the visual clue of the line segments and (B) concentration c_2 versus z-coordinate at selected line segments.

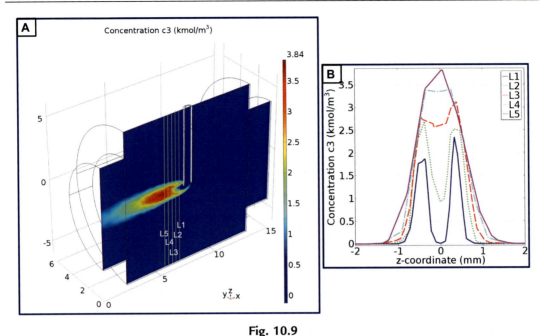

Fig. 10.9
Simulation of reacting species: (A) slice plot of the concentration c_3, (B) concentration c_3 versus z-coordinate at selected line segments.

The concentration c_3 of the reacting nanofluid with blood species is simulated in Fig. 10.9A. There is an abrupt rise in concentration after leaving from inlets but then starts to decrease with increasing distance from the point of injection. For quantitative analysis, we have selected the line segments whose visual clue is shown in Fig. 10.9A and the corresponding line plots along these line segments are shown in Fig. 10.9B. The species initially moves with parabolic order and then splits into the two branches and combined again with increasing distance from the point of injection.

Finally, we have simulated the total rate expression for three concentration species as demonstrated in Fig. 10.10. The simulation results show that the reaction rates for concentrations c_1 and c_2 are identical but the reaction rate for concentration c_3 is symmetrically opposite about $x=0$ axes. When reaction rates of concentrations c_1 and c_2 decreases, the reaction rate of concentration c_3 increases, and vice versa.

10.7 Conclusions

The reacting flow is almost homogenous in the porous part of the tissue. Therefore, the velocity at the center is maximum. The concentration c_1 of nanofluid decreases rapidly as its distance increases from the point of injection. This implies that porous tissue is not optimally used.

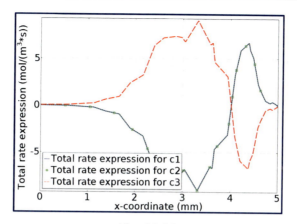

Fig. 10.10
Simulation of reaction rates versus x-coordinate.

For the concentration of blood species c_2, the reaction is not uniformly distributed in the porous medium and has a maximum close to the radial position of the injecting point. The concentration c_3 rises abruptly after leaving from inlets but as the distance increases from the point of injection, it starts to decrease again. The reaction rates for concentrations c_1 and c_2 are almost identical but the reaction rate for concentration c_3 is symmetrically opposite to c_2 and c_3 about $x=0$ axes. When reaction rates of concentrations c_1 and c_2 increases, the reaction rate of concentration c_3 decreases, and vice versa.

References

[1] Mackay DM, Freyberg D, Roberts P, Cherry J. A natural gradient experiment on solute transport in a sand aquifer: 1. Approach and overview of plume movement. Water Resour Res 1986;22:2017–29.
[2] Fetter CW, Boving T, Kreamer D. Contaminant hydrogeology. Waveland Press; 2017.
[3] Bear J, Verruijt A. Modeling groundwater flow and pollution. Springer Science & Business Media; 2012.
[4] Bear J. Hydraulics of groundwater. Courier Corporation; 2012.
[5] Daus AD, Frind EO. An alternating direction Galerkin technique for simulation of contaminant transport in complex groundwater systems. Water Resour Res 1985;21(5):653–64.
[6] Bear J. Dynamics of fluids in porous media. Courier Corporation; 2013.
[7] Millington R, Quirk J. Permeability of porous solids. Trans Faraday Soc 1961;57:1200–7.
[8] Buongiorno J. Convective transport in nanofluids. J Heat Transf 2006;128:240–50.
[9] Banerjee RK, van Osdol WW, Bungay PM, Sung C, Dedrick RL. Finite element model of antibody penetration in a prevascular tumor nodule embedded in normal tissue. J Control Release 2001;74:193–202.
[10] Graff CP, Wittrup KD. Theoretical analysis of antibody targeting of tumor spheroids: importance of dosage for penetration, and affinity for retention. Cancer Res 2003;63:1288–96.
[11] Kwok C, Yu S, Lee S. Mathematical models of the uptake kinetics of antitumor antibodies in human melanoma spheroids. Antib Immunoconjug Radiopharm 1995;8:155–69.
[12] Wenning LA, Murphy RM. Coupled cellular trafficking and diffusional limitations in delivery of immunotoxins to multicell tumor spheroids. Biotechnol Bioeng 1999;62:562–75.
[13] Goodman TT, Chen J, Matveev K, Pun SH. Spatio-temporal modeling of nanoparticle delivery to multicellular tumor spheroids. Biotechnol Bioeng 2008;101:388–99.

[14] Waite CL, Roth CM. Binding and transport of PAMAM-RGD in a tumor spheroid model: the effect of RGD targeting ligand density. Biotechnol Bioeng 2011;108:2999–3008.

[15] Al-Waeli AH, Chaichan MT, Kazem HA, Sopian K, Safaei J. Numerical study on the effect of operating nanofluids of photovoltaic thermal system (PV/T) on the convective heat transfer. Case Stud Therm Eng 2018;12:405–13.

[16] Brinkman H. A calculation of the viscous force exerted by a flowing fluid on a dense swarm of particles. Flow Turbul Combust 1949;1:27.

[17] Jacob M, Chappell D, Becker BF. Regulation of blood flow and volume exchange across the microcirculation. Crit Care 2016;20:319.

[18] Audigier C, Mansi T, Delingette H, Rapaka S, Mihalef V, Carnegie D, et al. Parameter estimation for personalization of liver tumor radiofrequency ablation. In: International MICCAI workshop on computational and clinical challenges in abdominal imaging. Springer; 2014. p. 3–12.

[19] Zohdi T, Kuypers F, Lee W. Estimation of red blood cell volume fraction from overall permittivity measurements. Int J Eng Sci 2010;48:1681–91.

CHAPTER 11

Thermal therapy of cylindrical tumor with optimization using Nelder-Mead method

Magnetic fluid hyperthermia (MFH) is a therapeutic procedure where the temperature of the tumor burdened with magnetic nanoparticles (MNPs) is elevated to 41–46°C when excited by the external applied magnetic field (AMF) [1]. The heat released by the MNPs under Neel and Brownian relaxation effects kill the tumor cells with minimum side effects [2]. During this procedure, special coils are utilized to generate a magnetic field of required intensity [3]. Mostly, the coils are in helical shape that surrounds the tumor tissue embedded with the MNPs [4]. The fundamental principles and practical application of induction heating appeared at the beginning of the 20th century. It took a major breakthrough during World War II and the postwar years [5]. This technology gradually paved its way to the medical society when used in MFH [6]. The basic purpose of a coil in MFH is to provide a constant AMF at a specific frequency. This AMF induces heating in the sample placed within this coil [7]. The magnetic energy from the coil depends on electrical conductivity, magnetic anisotropy, magnetization, field frequency, and magnetic intensity [8]. Different coil geometries are used in MFH including Helmholtz, birdcage, pancake, and solenoid. The most popular is the solenoidal coil because it is capable of handling currents and frequencies required in MFH processes [9].

11.1 Materials and methods

In this section, we will deal with the basic material properties and methodology used in our simulation study.

11.2 Nanofluid and its properties

The nanofluid in the current study consists of Fe_3O_4 MNPs of size 19 nm with the base fluid octane. The properties of nanofluid include volume fraction of 0.2127, density 1665 kg m^{-3}, heat capacity 388.40 J kg^{-1} K^{-1}, thermal conductivity 0.1825 W m^{-1} K^{-1}, and viscosity of nanofluid 9.27×10^{-4} Pa s. The details of calculations and theoretical formulas used for calculating these properties are shown in Appendix B.

11.3 Mathematical modeling formulation of the problem

To simulate the MFD developed by the current-carrying coil and associated heat generation in cancerous tissue, we will use the induction model. This model carries the basic equations that deal with our problem. All the involved models with ICs and BCs are demonstrated below.

11.3.1 Magnetic flux density developed by a multiturn coil

To simulate the magnetic flux density (MFD) developed by the current-carrying coil and associated heat generation in cancerous tissue, we will use the induction model. This model carries the basic equations that deal with our problem. All the involved models with ICs and BCs are demonstrated below. The coil generates magnetic field which coupled with Ampere's law is formulated as

$$\left.\begin{array}{r} \nabla \times \underline{H}_M = \underline{J}_e \\ \nabla \times (\mu_0^{-1}\mu_r^{-1}\underline{B}_M) = \sigma \underline{v} \times \underline{B}_M + \underline{J}_e \\ \underline{B}_M = \nabla \times \underline{A} \end{array}\right\} \quad (11.1)$$

where electric field and magnetic field are defined as $B_e = \mu_0\mu_r E_e$, $D_e = \varepsilon_0\varepsilon_r E_e$, where ε_0 and ε_r are permeability of free space and relative permeability, respectively, and μ_0 and μ_r are the permittivity of free space and relative permittivity, respectively. The magnetic insulation is defined as $n \times A = 0$, where n represents normal vector and $A = (0,0,0)$ Wb/m is the initial value of magnetic vector potential. The multiturn coil with N number of turns and A, as an area of cross section, is formulated as $J_e = (NI_{coil}/A)\ e_{coil}$, where I_{coil} is the coil current.

11.3.2 Steady-state analysis of bioheat transfer in liver tissue

Before switching on magnetic field for heat generation, we assumed that the nanofluid is distributed throughout the liver tissue after injecting the nanofluid in the tumor with a needle of size 15-gauge whose dimensions are described in Appendix A. After heat dissipation by the MNPs due to the application of the magnetic field, the heat transfers in the tumor interstitium. The transfer of heat in the liver tumor tissue is formulated by steady-state PBHTM [10] defined below. Using this model, the temperature can be predicted quantitatively in the liver tissue:

$$k\nabla^2 T + \omega_b\rho_b c_b(T_b - T) + Q_{met} + Q_{np} = 0, \quad Q_{np} = \pi\mu_0 H_0^2 f_0 \chi'' \quad (11.2)$$

where k, T, ω_b, ρ_b, c_b, T_b, and Q_m, are thermal conductivity of tissue, tissue temperature, local blood perfusion rate, the density of blood, specific heat capacity of blood, blood temperature, and metabolic heat generation rate, respectively. Q_{np} is the heat dissipation by MNPs based on

Rosensweig formulation [11], and for Fe_3O_4 MNPs, Q_{np} is calculated to be 3.33×10^5 W m^3. The details of all calculations involved are given in Appendix B. Without the heat term Q_{np}. The initial temperature in both normal and tumor tissues is taken as $T_0 = 37°C$. The outer boundary of normal tissue is experiencing convective heat flux condition, $-n(-k\nabla T) = h(T_{ext} - T)$ where $h = 200$ W/K/m^2 is the heat transfer coefficient and $T_{ext} = 37°C$.

11.3.3 Analytical solution of steady-state bioheat transfer model

The steady-state heat transfer model Eq. (11.2) can be written in cylindrical coordinates as

$$k\frac{1}{r}\frac{d}{dr}\left(r\frac{dT}{dr}\right) + \omega_b \rho_b c_b (T_b - T) + Q_{met} = 0 \quad (11.3)$$

With the term Q_{np}, the above equation becomes

$$k\frac{1}{r}\frac{d}{dr}\left(r\frac{dT}{dr}\right) + \omega_b \rho_b c_b (T_b - T) + (Q_{met} + Q_{np}) = 0 \quad (11.4)$$

The analytical solution of the above equation with the aid of solution by Yue et al. [12] is given by

$$T(r^*) = T_\infty + (T_a + T_\infty)\left(1 + \frac{(Q_m^* + Q_{np}^*)}{\omega_b^*}\right)\left[1 - \frac{I_0\left(\sqrt{\omega_b^*}r\right)}{I_0\left(\sqrt{\omega_b^*}\right) + \frac{\sqrt{\omega_b^*}}{h_A^*}I_1\left(\sqrt{\omega_b^*}\right)}\right] \quad (11.5)$$

where $h_A^* = h_A R/K$, $r^* = r/R$, $\omega_b^* = \omega_b c_b R^2/K$, and $Q_m^* = Q_m R^2/k(T_a - T_\infty)$. The Bessel functions of first and second-order up to third terms are given by

$$\begin{aligned} I_0(x) &= 1 - \frac{x^2}{2^2(1)^2} + \frac{x^4}{2^4(1)^2} - \frac{x^6}{2^6(1)^2} \\ I_1(x) &= \frac{x}{2} - \frac{x^3}{2^3 12} + \frac{x^5}{2^5 23} - \frac{x^7}{2^7 34} \end{aligned} \quad (11.6)$$

Using above functions, we get

$$\begin{aligned} I_0\left(\sqrt{\omega_b^*}\right) &= 1 - 6 \times 10^3 R^2 + 9 \times 10^6 R^4 \\ I_0\left(\sqrt{\omega_b^*}r^*\right) &= 1 - 6 \times 10^3 r^2 + 9 \times 10^6 r^4 \\ I_1\left(\sqrt{\omega_b^*}\right) &= 77.56R - 2 \times 10^5 R^3 + 2 \times 10^8 R^5 \end{aligned} \quad (11.7)$$

The analytical solution becomes

$$T\left(\frac{r}{R}\right) = 298 + 40.92\left[1 - \frac{(1 - 6 \times 10^3 r^2 + 9 \times 10^6 r^4)}{(1 - 6 \times 10^3 R^2 + 9 \times 10^6 R^4) + 7.4291(77.56R - 2 \times 10^5 R^3 + 2 \times 10^8 R^5)}\right] \tag{11.8}$$

where R is the radius of liver tissue and r is radial coordinate, and the remaining values used are as follows:

$$h_A^* = 20.88R, \quad \omega_b^* = 24062.5, \quad \frac{\sqrt{\omega_b^*}}{h_A^*} = 7.4291, \quad \frac{Q_m^* + Q_{np}^*}{\omega_b^*} = 2.4104 \tag{11.9}$$

11.3.4 Transient analytical of bioheat transfer in liver tissue

For time-dependent analysis we have incorporated the heat dissipation by MNPs into time-dependent PBHTM, the model is demonstrated below, where all terms have already been defined in the model (14.10):

$$\rho C_p \frac{\partial T}{\partial t} = k\nabla^2 T + \omega_b \rho_b c_b(T_b - T) + Q_{met} + Q_{np}, \quad Q_{np} = \pi\mu_0 H_0^2 f_0 \chi'' \tag{11.10}$$

11.3.5 Construction of optimization problem model

Next, we have constructed our optimization problem as

$$\begin{aligned} &\min |T_{sim} - T_{exp}|^2 \\ &\text{Subject to} \\ &0.1 \leq k \leq 3 \end{aligned} \tag{11.11}$$

where T_{sim} and T_{exp} represent simulated and experimental temperatures, respectively. The objective is to minimize the error between these two temperatures through the best fitting. The squared term represents the positive factor. The control variable is thermal conductivity, $0.1 \leq k \leq 3$. We will use the Nelder-Mead optimization method to minimize the objective developed in our formulated problem. The detailed algorithm of the Nelder-Mead method can be found in Ref. [13].

11.3.6 Adding physics, studies, and geometry construction of the problem

From the model wizard, a 3D space dimension is selected and the physics for the problem is selected as *magnetic field* and *bioheat heat transfer* model. Both physics are coupled through Multiphysics coupling. The study for the both physics has been added as stationary for steady-state analysis. After adding the physics and corresponding studies to the problem, the geometry of the problem is constructed. The length units of the geometry are selected in mm and angular units are selected in degrees. Four concentric cylinders are constructed with the dimensions as shown in Table 11.1.

11.3.7 Adding a material, initial condition, and boundary conditions

The material for domain 1 and domain 2 is added as liver because we are dealing with liver tumor tissue. The material for domain 3 is added as copper because we are considering a multiturn coil composed of copper. The material for domain 4 is added as air because it acts as

Table 11.1 Dimensions of objects in the geometry of the problem.

Object type	Radius (mm)	Height (mm)	Position (x,y,z)	Axis
Cylinder 1	5	30	(0,0,5)	z-axis
Cylinder 2	15	30	(0,0,5)	z-axis
Cylinder 3	30	40	(0,0,0)	z-axis
Cylinder 4	50	40	(0,0,0)	z-axis

Cylinder 1, cylinder 2, cylinder 3, and cylinder 4 are labeled as domain 1 (tumor tissue), domain 2 (healthy tissue), domain 3 (multiturn coil), and domain 4 (external air domain), respectively. The whole geometry with all domains is shown in Fig. 11.1.

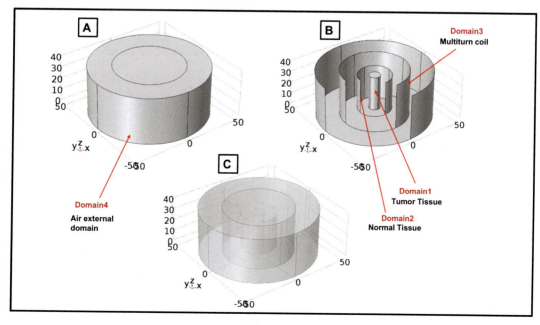

Fig. 11.1
Geometry of the model (A) domain 4 surrounding domain 3, domain 2, and domain 1, (B) each domain labeled representing coil, healthy tissue, and tumor tissue, and (C) transparent view of whole geometry.

an external domain. The properties of added materials air, copper, and liver are demonstrated in Tables 11.2–11.5.

The IC for the coil was added as a magnetic vector potential $A=(0,0,0)$ Wb/m whereas the IC for the liver was added as initial temperature $T=310.15$ K. Since we are dealing with a multiturn coil, we have inserted $n=100$ as the number of coil turns and coil current as 400 A [15]. The reference edge for this multiturn coil is shown in Fig. 11.2A. The corresponding heat source in liver tissue is shown in Fig. 11.2B where the value of Q_{np} as 3.33×10^5 Wm^{-3} is inserted. The convective flux boundary condition for liver healthy tissue is added as shown in Fig. 11.2C. The parameters involved in the biological tissue are added as shown in Table 11.2.

11.3.8 Mesh generation of the model

After adding physics, corresponding studies, materials, ICs, and BCs, the mesh of the model is generated in different mesh modes as shown in Fig. 11.3. The details of different meshes is documented in Table 11.6.

Table 11.2 Material properties of Air (Built-in COMSOL).

Electrical conductivity	Relative permeability	Relative permittivity	Refractive index	The ratio of specific heats	Refractive index image. Part
0 S m^{-1}	1 1	1 1	1 1	1.4 1	0 1

Table 11.3 Material properties of Copper (Built-in COMSOL).

Thermal conductivity	Relative permeability	Relative permittivity	Electrical conductivity	Heat capacity at constant pressure	Density
400 Wm^{-1} K^{-1}	1 1	1 1	5.998×10^7 S m^{-1}	385 J kg^{-1} K^{-1}	8700 kg m^{-3}

Table 11.4 Material properties of Liver (Built-in COMSOL).

Heat capacity at constant pressure	Thermal conductivity	Relative permittivity	Electrical conductivity	Relative permeability	Density
3450 J kg^{-1} K^{-1}	0.52 Wm^{-1} K^{-1}	1 1	0.52 Sm^{-1}	1 1	1079 kg m^{-3}

Table 11.5 Physical properties of the liver [14].

Tissue	Density (kg/m^3)	Heat capacity (J/kg/°C)	Thermal conductivity (Wm^{-1}/°C)	Heat transfer rate (mL/min/kg)	Heat generation rate (W/kg)
Liver	1079	3540	0.52	860	9.93

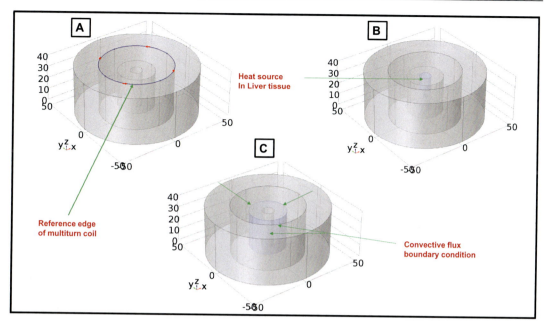

Fig. 11.2
Adding boundary conditions to the corresponding physics and heat source to the liver tissue.

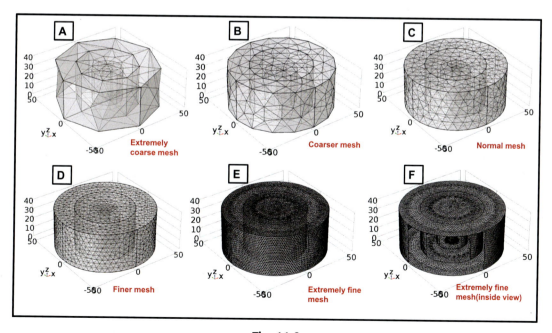

Fig. 11.3
Mesh generation of the model: Mesh consists of tetrahedral elements (A) mesh in extremely coarse mode, (B) mesh in coarser mode, (C) mesh in normal mode, (D) mesh in finer mode, (E) mesh in extremely fine mode, and (F) mesh with an inside view.

Table 11.6 Mesh analysis of the model.

Mesh type	Number of vertex elements	Number of edge elements	Number of boundary elements	Number of elements	Free meshing time(s)	Minimum element quality
Extremely coarse	32	0120	00448	001151	00.25	0.03666
Coarser	32	0168	00880	002685	00.45	0.04807
Normal	32	0252	01864	008542	00.56	0.05453
Finer	32	0412	04644	037426	01.77	0.10820
Extremely fine	32	1012	27,770	682,774	17.62	0.17050

11.4 Results

We have firstly simulated the magnetic field generated by the current-carrying coil and the resulting MFD is shown in Fig. 11.4A. Maximum MFD of 0.97 Tesla (T) is reached. The coil is carrying a current of $I_{coil} = 400 A$ and it has 100 turns. The MFD is well distributed throughout the model domains. The arrow plot of MFD is simulated in Fig. 11.4B. Showing the direction of magnetic field lines following the right-hand rule where the current flowing in the coil with the

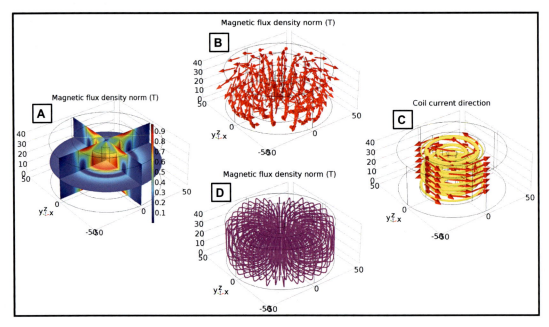

Fig. 11.4
Simulation of the magnetic field generated by current-carrying coil: (A) MFD distribution, (B) MFD with arrow plot, (C) coil current direction, and (D) streamline plot of the MFD.

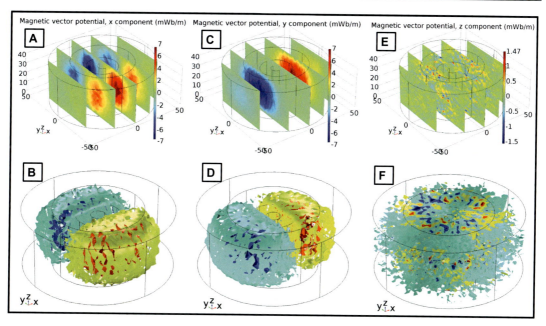

Fig. 11.5

Simulation of magnetic vector potential: (A) A_x component of the magnetic vector potential, (B) the isosurface plot of A_x component (C) A_y component of the magnetic vector potential, (D) the isosurface plot of A_y component, (E) A_z component of the magnetic vector potential, and (F) the isosurface plot of A_x component.

direction of fingers of your right hand then the thumb will be in an upward direction as shown in Fig. 11.4C. Streamline plot of MFD is also added in Fig. 11.4D where MFD is crossing well the axial location of the coil, which is our objective to heat liver tumor located at the axially centric location of the coil.

The simulation of the magnetic vector potential involved in the electrodynamics of model (2) is demonstrated in Fig. 11.5. The x-component of the magnetic vector potential A_x is shown in Fig. 11.5A. The distribution of A_x is maximum in the region $y<0$ and A_x is more concentrated in this region as compared to the region $y>0$ where the distribution of A_x is minimum. The corresponding isosurface is simulated in Fig. 11.5B. The y-component of the magnetic vector potential A_y is shown in Fig. 11.5C. The distribution of A_y is maximum in the region $x>0$ and A_y is more concentrated in this region as compared to the region $x<0$ where the distribution of A_y is minimum. To visualize, the corresponding isosurface is simulated in Fig. 11.5D. The z-component of the magnetic vector potential A_z is shown in Fig. 11.5E. The distribution of A_z is contrary to A_x and A_y, it is mixed with maximum and minimum values. To visualize, corresponding isosurface is simulated in Fig. 11.5F. The maximum values of A_x and A_y are nearly equal to 7mWb/m and minimum values −7mWb/m. The A_z component gets a maximum

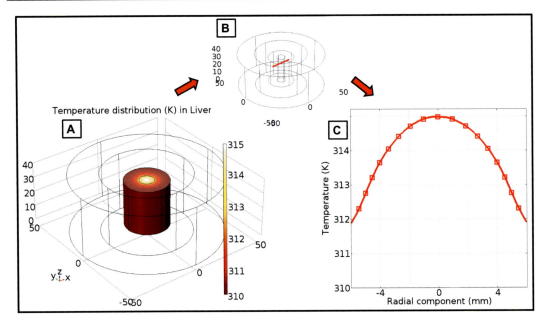

Fig. 11.6

Simulation of steady-state temperature distribution in the liver tissue: (A) 3D temperature distribution in liver tissue, (B) visual clue of selected line segment, and (C) temperature versus radial axis profile along arclength.

potential of 1.47 mWb/m and a minimum of −1.5 mWb/m. Thus, the electromagnetic potential distribution covers more regions along the *x*-axis and *y*-axis and covers less space along the *z*-axis.

Next, we have a simulated model (14.2) for steady-state analysis. The temperature distribution produced due to heat generation by vibrating MNPs under the influence of the coil magnetic field in liver tissue is simulated in Fig. 11.6A. The temperature is elevated to 315 K from the normal temperature of the body. For quantitative analysis, we have selected line segments as shown in Fig. 11.6B, and temperature versus radial axis along these line segments is shown in Fig. 11.6C. The temperature at the tumor center is maximum and it decreases as we move radially outward.

We have simulated the analytical model (14.8) for temperature versus radial distance. The comparison of the analytical curve with the simulated temperature curve for steady-state analysis is shown in Fig. 11.7. This shows good agreement of simulation results with analytical results.

The time-dependent solution of bioheat transfer is shown in Fig. 11.8A. The maximum temperature is obtained at the center of the tumor and the minimum at the outer edges of the tumor. For quantitative analysis, we have selected six points P_i: $i = 1 \leq i \leq 6$. The visual clue of

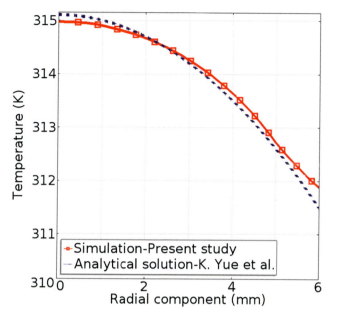

Fig. 11.7
Comparison of analytical and simulated curves.

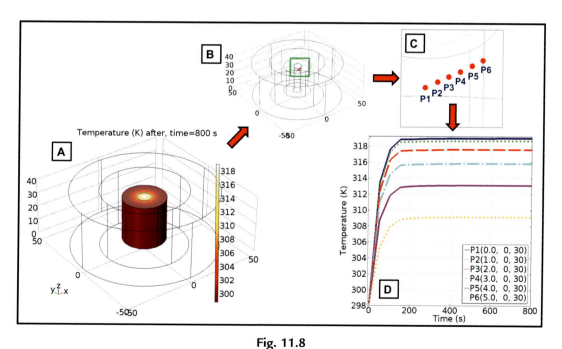

Fig. 11.8
Transient analysis of liver tissue heating, (A) temperature distribution in liver tissue, (B) visual clue of selected points, (C) zoomed view of selected points, and (D) temperature versus time curves at selected points.

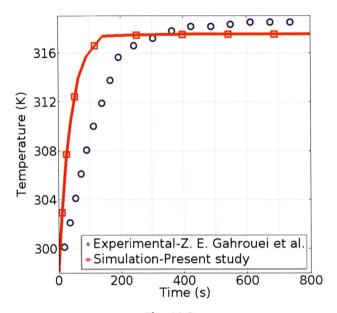

Fig. 11.9
Optimized fitting of the simulated curve with the experimental curve.

these selected points is shown in Fig. 11.8B, the zoomed view of selected points is shown in Fig. 11.8C. The corresponding temperature versus time profiles are shown in Fig. 11.8D. The results show that with time, the temperature increases and after reaching a maximum temperature within first 15 min, the temperature reaches a steady-state. Moreover, the temperature at the point P_1 is higher than any other point at the specific time. This result shows that temperature at the center of the tumor is higher which is required in our problem for best heating which will ultimately destroy tumor cells effectively at this elevated temperature. For transient analysis, we have taken the base temperature to be 298 K because the experimental data for which we are going to perform optimization was available in this range.

Next, we have simulated the optimization problem based on the least-square objective. We have run our optimization problem and our simulated curve gave the best-optimized fit with experimental data for thermal conductivity of 0.1426 Wm^{-1} K^{-1} as shown in Fig. 11.9. The experiential data is taken from the study by Gahrouei et al. [16]. They dealt with MFH experimentally for transient analysis.

11.5 Conclusions

The MFD generated from the current-carrying solenoidal coil is simulated in three dimensions. The direction of current in the coil is anticlockwise and magnetic field lines are in an upward direction following the right-hand rule. The magnetic vector potential is simulated along the three coordinate axes and its distribution is not the same in all three coordinate axis directions. The distribution of the z component of magnetic vector potential is a uniformly mixed distribution contrary to x and y components that were maximum in one half region and minimum in the other half region. The induction of the magnetic field with the liver tumor surrounded by the normal tissue generates steady-state heat in the tumor tissue for tumor cell damage. The temperature distribution inside the tumor has been predicted quantitatively and maximum temperature is obtained at the tumor center and minimum at the outer edge of the tumor. The transient analysis of the tumor heating resulted in increasing temperature with the passage of heating time. The optimization problem is constructed subject to constraint. The transient temperature versus time curve is optimized for the best fit using the Nelder-Mead method. A good fitting was achieved for the thermal conductivity $k=0.1426\,\mathrm{W\,m^{-1}K^{-1}}$. In the future, we are interested to optimize MFD to achieve efficient tumor heating.

References

[1] Deatsch AE, Evans BA. Heating efficiency in magnetic nanoparticle hyperthermia. J Magn Magn Mater 2014;354:163–72.

[2] Hergt R, Andra W, d'Ambly CG, Hilger I, Kaiser WA, Richter U, et al. Physical limits of hyperthermia using magnetite fine particles. IEEE Trans Magn 1998;34:3745–54.

[3] Miaskowski A, Sawicki B, Subramanian M. Single-domain nanoparticle magnetic power losses calibrated with calorimetric measurements. Bull Pol Acad Sci Tech Sci 2018;66.

[4] Gas P, Miaskowski A. Specifying the ferrofluid parameters important from the viewpoint of magnetic fluid hyperthermia. In: 2015 selected problems of electrical engineering and electronics (WZEE). IEEE; 2015. p. 1–6.

[5] Bates L. Some post-war developments in magnetism. Proc Phys Soc Sect A 1952;65:577.

[6] Perigo EA, Hemery G, Sandre O, Ortega D, Garaio E, Plazaola F, et al. Fundamentals and advances in magnetic hyperthermia. Appl Phys Rev 2015;2, 041302.

[7] Ortega D, Pankhurst QA. Magnetic hyperthermia. Nanoscience 2013;1, e88.

[8] Tong S, Quinto CA, Zhang L, Mohindra P, Bao G. Size-dependent heating of magnetic iron oxide nanoparticles. ACS Nano 2017;11:6808–16.

[9] Cabrera D, Rubia-Rodríguez I, Garaio E, Plazaola F, Dupré L, Farrow N, et al. Instrumentation for magnetic hyperthermia. In: Nanomaterials for magnetic and optical hyperthermia applications. Elsevier; 2019. p. 111–38.

[10] Pennes HH. Analysis of tissue and arterial blood temperatures in the resting human forearm. J Appl Physiol 1948;1:93–122.

[11] Rosensweig RE. Heating magnetic fluid with alternating magnetic field. J Magn Magn Mater 2002;252:370–4.

[12] Yue K, Zhang X, Yu F. An analytic solution of one-dimensional steady-state Pennes' bioheat transfer equation in cylindrical coordinates. J Therm Sci 2004;13:255–8.

[13] Nelder JA, Mead R. A simplex method for function minimization. Comput J 1965;7:308–13.

[14] Hasgall P, Di Gennaro F, Baumgartner C, Neufeld E, Lloyd B, Gosselin M, et al. IT'IS Database for thermal and electromagnetic parameters of biological tissues, 2018. Version 4.0, May 15, 2018. 10.13099. VIP21000–04-0. Onl www.itis.ethz.ch/database.

[15] Miaskowski A, Sawicki B, Krawczyk A, Yamada S. The application of magnetic fluid hyperthermia to breast cancer treatment. Electr Rev 2010;86:99–101.

[16] Galmouci ZE, Labhaf S, Kermanpur A. Cobalt doped magnetite nanoparticles: synthesis, characterization, optimization and suitability evaluations for magnetic hyperthermia applications. Physica E 2020;116, 113759.

Supplementary material: Appendix A

Supplementary material: In silico study of hyperthermia of Liver cancer using CoFe2O4@MnFe2O4 MNPs

Color code:
- Input
- Dependent on output
- Not used
- Biometric

	Formula	Value 1	Units	Value 2	Units	Reference or link
Dimensions of needle						
Needle outer diameter, Do		1.829	mm	15	Ga	https://en.wikipedia.org/wiki/Birmingham_gauge
Needle inner diameter, Di		1.372	mm			https://en.wikipedia.org/wiki/Birmingham_gauge
Needle outer radius, ro	Do/2	0.915	mm			
Needle inner radius, ri	Di/2	0.686	mm	6.86E-04	m	
Needle wall thickness, d	ro-ri	0.23	mm			
Flux of nanofluid						
Volumetric flow rate, ς		3	µL/min	5E-11	m³/s	
Inner area = needle area, Ai	π^*r^2	1.48E+06	m²			
Density of MNP, ρmp		5300	kg/m³			https://www.aqua-calc.com/page/density-table/substance/tailinic
Density of base fluid, ρw		2170	kg/m³			
Volume fraction on MNP, φ		0.0013				
Density of nanofluid, ρnf	ρmp*φ+ρw*(1-φ)	2174	kg/m³			
Flux of nanofluid	ς*ρnf/Ai	7.33E-02	kg/s/m²	2.10E-03	mol/h/cm²	
Molar mass of core+shell	%Vc*Mc+%Vs*Ms	231.5	g/mol			
Molar mass of nanoparticles						
Molar mass of core CoFe2O4, Mc		234.6208	g/mol			https://en.snl.chemicalaid.com/tools/molarmass.php?formula=CoFe2O4
Molar mass of shell MnFe2O4, Ms		230.6296	g/mol			https://en.snl.chemicalaid.com/tools/molarmass.php?formula=MnFe2O4
Diameter of core, Dc		9	nm			
Volume of core, Vc	(4/3)*π*(Dc/2)³	382	nm³			
Diameter of shell, Ds		15	nm			
Volume of NP, Vnp	(4/3)*π*(Ds/2)³	1767	nm³			
Volume of shell MnFe2O4, Vs	Vnp-Vc	1385	nm³			
Ratio Vshell/Vcore	Vs/Vc	3.63				
% Vcore, %Vc	Vc/Vnp	22%				
% Vshell, %Vs	Vs/Vnp	78%				
Molar mass of NaCl		58.44	g/mol			
Molar mass of Water		18.01	g/mol			
Molar mass of Saline		76.45	g/mol			
Molar mass of nano fluid		307.94	g/mol			
Mass concentration						
Mass concentration ρnp	((fjmass/fluid)	2.85	kg/m³	0.573659856	mol/m³	
Diffusion coefficient, Di						
Boltzmann constant, kB		1.38E-23	J/K			
Absolute temperature, T		310.15	K			
Hydrodynamics volume of NP, vh		8.84E-06	Pa·s			
Dynamic viscosity of water, η		1.22E+00	cP			
Dynamic viscosity of NaCl, η		1.25E-03	Pa·s			
Dynamic viscosity of nanofluid saline, η		1.23E-03	Pa·s	7.5E-09	m	https://www.omi.gov/acrv/tahwar/0521414
Radius of nanoparticle, rp		7.5	nm			
Diffusion coefficient, Di	(kBT ε(6πηrp)	2.46E-11	m²/s			3.1837E-07
Heat dissipation, Qnp						
Diameter of NP, D		15	nm	1.5E-08	m	
Legand layer thickness, δ		1	nm	1E-09	m	
Volume of nanoparticle, vm	(p/4)*D³/6	1.7664E+24	m³			
Hydrodynamics volume of NP, vh	(p/4)*(2*delta)³/6	2.571E+24	m³			
Magnetic field intensity, H0		2.65	kA/m	2650	A/m	
Frequency of magnetic field, f0		500	kHz	500000	Hz	
Angular frequency, ω	2πf0	3.141000	Hz	0.000318371	m	
Time of heating, t0		60	min	3600	s	
Product1		1.91012E-05				
Product2		1130760000000				
Magnetic field, H	H0*cos(omega*t0)	2650	A/m			
Domain magnetization of suspended NP, Md		6.30E+05	A/m			
volume fraction, fi		0.0013				
Permeability of free space, μ0		1.2564E-06	H/m			
Boltzmann constant, kB	4*pi*1e-7	1.38E-23	J/K			
Absolute temperature, T0		310.15	K			
Magnetic anisotropy constant, K		1.50E+04	J/m³			
Brownian relaxation time, τb	(3*vp*n)/(k+βT0)	2.22E-06				
Gamma, Γ	(K*vm)/(kB*T0)	6.19E+03				
Average relaxation time, τ0		1.00E-09	s			
Neel relaxation time, τN	(sqrt(pi/2)*tau0*exp(Gamma)/sqrt(Gamma))	1.74E-07				
Relaxation time, τ	(tau0*tauB)/(tauN+tauB)	1.61E-07				
ωτ, ξ	(mu0*M0*H*H*vm)(kB*T0)	8.74E-03				
γ0		9.09E-02				
γ0'	X(1+tau*tau0)/cos(tau+1/(tau+1))	8.60E-02				
Qnp	p*mu0*X0*(H0^2/2*f0*(omega*tau/(1+omega*tau^2))	4.81E+05	W/m³			

Supplementary material: Appendix B

Supplementary data: In silico study of magnetic fluid hyperthermia of poroelastic brain tumor

Color code:
- Input
- Dependent on output
- Not used
- Remarks

Parameters	Formula	Value 1	Units	Value 2	Units	Reference or link	Remarks
Dimensions of needle							
Needle outer diameter, Do		1.829	mm	15	Ga	https://en.wikipedia.org/wiki/Birmingham_gauge	
Needle inner diameter, Di		1.372	mm			https://en.wikipedia.org/wiki/Birmingham_gauge	
Needle outer radius, ro	Do/2	0.915	mm				
Needle inner radius, ri	Di/2	0.686	mm	6.86E-04	m		
Needle wall thickness, d	ro-ri	0.23	mm				
Flow of nanofluid							
Volumetric flow rate, V		3	μL/min				
Inner area = needle area, Ai	π*ri²	1.48E-06	m²	1E-11	m³/s		
Density MNP, ρnp		3890	kg/m³				
Volume fraction on MNP, φ	((C19/C12)/((C19/C12)+(C20/C13)))*100%	997.1	kg/m³			https://www.aqua-calc.com/page/density-table/substance/saline	
Density of base fluid, ρw		0.043225493					
Density of nanofluid, ρnf	ρnp*φ + ρw*(1-φ)	3996	kg/m³				
Flux of nanofluid,	V*nf/Ai	1.02E-01	kg/s/m²	1.72E-01	mol/s/m²		
Molar mass of nanoparticles							
Molar mass of core Fe3O4, Mc		159.687	g/mol				
Molar mass of water, Mw		18.02	g/mol				
Molar mass of mass fluid		197.71	g/mol	0.17707	kg/mol		
Mass concentration							
Mass concentration ynp	ff*ρnanofluid	2086+04	kg/m³	1.17E+3555	mol/m3		
Diffusion coefficient, Di							
Boltzmann constant, kB		1.38E-23	J/K				
Absolute temperature, T		310.15	K				
Dynamic viscosity of water, η		8.90E-01	cP				
Radius of nanoparticle, rp		8.90E-04	Pa s	7.5E-09	m	http://www.cge.ugg.com/wien/data/v31c14	
Diffusion coefficient, Di	(kBT)/(6πηrp)	7.5	nm				
		1.76E-12	m2/s				
Heat dissipation, Qnp							
Diameter of NP, Di		15	nm	1.5E-08	m		
Legend layer thickness, δ		1	nm	1E-09	m		
volume of nanoparticle, vm	(p*D^3)/6	1.7668E-24	m³				
Hydrodynamics volume of NP, vh	(p*(D+2*delta)^3)/6	2.5714E-24	m³				
Magnetic field intensity, H0		2.65	kA/m	2650	A/m		
Permeability of magnetic field, f0		500	kHz	500000	Hz		
Frequency of magnetic field, f0		314000	Hz				
Angular frequency, ω	2πf0	3141000	Hz	0.00031837	ms	3.1837E-07	s
Time of heating, t0		60	ms	3600	s		
Product1	ω*t0	1.91022E-05	-				
Product2	ω*t0						
Product3	H0²cos(omega*t0)						
Magnetic field, H		11307600000					
Domain magnetization of suspended NP, Md	(np*(p)/2)*mu^0*(exp(Gamma)/sqrt(Gamma))	2650	A/m	1.5E-08	A/m		
Volume fraction, fv	(mu^0*vm)/(kB*T*tau)	6.36E+05	A/m	1E-09			
Permeability of free space, μ0	4*pi*1e-7	0.0013					
Magnetic field intensity, kB		1.256E-06	H/m				
Boltzmann constant, kB		1.38E-23	J/K				
Absolute temperature, T0		310.15	K				
Magnetic anisotropy constant, K	(1*mu^0)/(kB*T0)	1.60E-06	J/m³				
Brownian relaxation time, τb	(K*vm)/(kB*T0)	5.10E+00	s				
Gamma, Γ		1.69E+00					
Average relaxation time, τ0	(sqrt(pi)/2)*mu^0*(exp(Gamma)/sqrt(Gamma))	1.74E+07					
Neel relaxation time, τN	(tau0*tauB)/(tau0+tauB)	1.57E-07					
Relaxation time, τ	(mu0*Md²*f*mu)/((kB*T0))	8.74E-01					
, τf	(mu0*Md²*f*mu)/((kB*T0))	9.69E-02					
, χ0	X^(1/tau)*(omega*(1+(omega*tau)/2))	1.60E-06	J/m³				
Qnp	p*mu0*X0*(H0^2)*f0*((omega*tau)/(1+(omega*tau)^2))	4.73E+05	W/m³				
Dynamic viscosity of nanofluid							
	ηnf=ηf(1-φ)^2.5	1.72E-02					
Specific heat capacity of nanofluid							
Specific heat capacity of water, Cw		4183	J/kg/C				
Specific heat capacity of Al2O3		765	J/kg/K				
Specific heat capacity of nanofluid	C12*C14-C13*(1-C14)	1809.795466	J/kg/K				
Specific heat capacity of blood		3500	J/kg/K				
Total specific heat capacity		5309.795466	J/kg/K				
Lame Constants							
Young modulus	E	0.5	MPa	5.00E+05	Pa		
Poisson's ratio	ν	0.35					
Bulk Modulus, K	Ev/((1+v)(1-2v))	432098.7654					
Shear Modulus, G	E/2(1+K)	0.578757009					

Supplementary material: Appendix C

Magnetic fluid hyperthermia of 2D female breast cancer

Parameter	Formula	Value 1	Units	Appendix C: Supplementary Material	Value 2	Units	Reference or link
Dimensions of needle							
Needle outer diameter, Do		1.829	mm				
Needle inner diameter, Di		1.372	mm				
Needle outer radius, ro	Do/2	0.915	mm				
Needle inner radius, ri	Di/2	0.686	mm				
Needle wall thickness, d	ro-ri	0.23	mm				
Flux of nanofluid							
Volumetric flow rate, V		3	μL/min		15	Gu	
Inner area = needle area, Ai	π*ri²	1.48E-06	m²				
Density MNP, ρnp		5300	kg/m³				
Density of base fluid, ρw		2170	kg/m³				
Volume Fraction on MNP, φ		0.0013	-		8.80E-04	m	
Density of nanofluid, ρnf	ρnp*(1-φ)+ρw*(1-φ)	2174	kg/m³				
flux of nanofluid	V*ρnf/Ai	7.35E-02	kg/s/m²		2.39E-03	mol/s/m²	
Molar mass of core+shell	%Vc*Mc+%Vs*Ms	231.5	g/mol				
Molar mass of nanoparticles							
Molar mass of core CoFe2O4, Mc		234.6208	g/mol				
Molar mass of shell MnFe2O4, Ms		230.6296	g/mol				
Diameter of core, Dc		9	nm				
Volume of core, Vc	(4/3)*π*(Dc/2)³	382	nm³				
Diameter of shell, Ds		15	nm				
Volume of NP, Vnp	(4/3)*π*(Ds/2)³	1767	nm³				
Volume of shell MnFe2O4, Vs	Vnp-Vc	1385	nm³				
Ratio Vshell/Vcore	Vs/Vc	3.63	-				
%Vcore, %Vc	Vc/Vnp	22%	-				
%Vshell, %Vs	Vs/Vnp	78%	-				
Molar mass of NaCl		58.44	g/mol				
Molar mass of Water		18.01	g/mol				
Molar mass of Saline		76.45	g/mol				

Parameter	Formula	Value 1	Units		Value 2	Units	Reference
Molar mass of nano fluid		107.94	g/mol		0.3079386	kg/mol	
Mass concentration	(f*ρnanofluid)	2.81	kg/m³		9.178096	mol/m3	
Boltzmann constant, kB		1.38E-23	J/K				
Absolute temperature, T		310.15	K				
Dynamic viscosity of water, η		8.90E-06	Pa·s				
Dynamic viscosity of NaCl, η		1.22E-03	cP				
Dynamic viscosity of nanofluid saline, η		1.22E-03	Pa·s				
Radius of nanoparticle, rp		7.5	nm		7.5E-09	m	
Diffusion coefficient, Di	(kBT)/(6πηrp)	2.46E-11	m²/s				
Dynamic viscosity of nanofluid	η0(1-φ)^2.5	1.23E-03	Pa·s				
Heat dissipation, Qpp							
Diameter of NP, Di		15	nm		1.5E-08	m	
Legend layer thickness, δ		1	nm		1E-09	m	
Volume of nanoparticles, v	(p*D³)/6	1.76E-24	m³				
Hydrodynamic volume of NP, vh	(p*(D+2*delta)³)/6	2.57E-24	m³				
Magnetic field intensity, H0		2.65	kA/m		2650	A/m	
Frequency of magnetic field, f0		500	kHz		500000	Hz	
Angular frequency, ω	2πf0	3.14E06	Hz		0.000318 4	m	3.1837E-07 s
Time of heating,t0		60			3600	s	
Product1	αβ	1.91922E+05					
Product2	αβ²	1.19276000000					
Magnetic field, H	H0*cos(omeg*t0)	2650	A/m				
Domain magnetization of suspended NP, Md		6.36E+05	A/m				
Volume Fraction, fl		0.0013	H/m				
Permeability of free space, μ0	4*pi*1e-7	1.2564E-6	H/m				
Boltzmann constant, kB		1.38E-23	J/K				
Absolute temperature, T0		310.15	K				
Magnetic anisotropy constant, K		1.50E+04	J/m³				
Brownian relaxation time, tb	(3*η*vh)/(kBT0)	2.22E-06	s				
Gamma, Γ	(K*vn)/(kBT0)	6.19E+00					
Average relaxation time, t0	(sqrt(pi)/2)*tau0*exp(Gamma)/sqrt(Gamma)	1.74E-07					
Neel relaxation time, tN	(tau*tau b)/(tau+tau b)	1.61E-07	s				
Relaxation time, τ		8.74E-01					
avi,ξ	(mu0*Md*H*pi*D³)/(6*kB*T0)	9.69E-02					
χ0	(mu0*f*Md²*pi*D³*vn)/(18*kB*T0)						

continued

Chp	$X(\Gamma3)xu)*(coth(xu)-1/(xu))$	8.60E-02	
Inflow velocity	$\mu*mu0*X0*(H0^2)*0*(omega*tau)/(1+(omega*tau)^2))$	4.84E+05	W/m^3
Flow rate	Q	3.00E-06	L/mn
Inflow velocity	v=Q/A	4.44E-12	

Quantitative analysis of MNPs size dependent heat dissipation

Size of nanoparticle	Heat dissipation
14	1.80E+05
15	4.83E+05
16	7.32E+05
17	5.57E+05
18	4.25E+05
19	3.80E+05

Heat dissipation (W/m^3) by MNPs of different sizes (nm)

- 14 nm: 1.80E+05
- 15 nm: 4.83E+05
- 16 nm: 7.32E+05
- 17 nm: 5.57E+05
- 18 nm: 4.25E+05
- 19 nm: 3.80E+05

Supplementary material: Appendix D

MFH of 3D Breast cancer therapy using Fe₃O₄ magnetic nanoparticles

Color code:
- Input (yellow)
- Dependent on output (blue/grey)
- Not used (red)
- Source (green)

Parameters	Formula	Value 1	Units	Value 2	Units	Reference or link
Dimensions of needle						
Needle outer diameter, Do		1.829	mm	15	Ga	https://www.uniquest.org.uk/lgb.needle_gauges
Needle inner diameter, Di		1.372	mm			https://www.sigmaaldrich.com/chemistry/stockroom-reagents/learning-center/technical-library/needle-gauge-chart.html
Needle outer radius, ro	Do/2	0.915	mm			
Needle inner radius, ri	Di/2	0.686	mm	8.8E-04	m	
Needle wall thickness, d	ro-ri	0.23	mm			
Flux of nanofluid						
Volumetric flow rate, V		3	μL/min	5E-11	m³/s	
Inner area = needle area, Ai	π*ri²	1.48E-06	m²			Javid et al (2014)
Density MNP, ρρp		5240	kg/m³			https://www.american-elements.com/iron-ii-iii-oxide-magnetic-nanoparticles-1317-61-9.html
Density of base fluid, ρw		698.6	kg/m³			Eq 1
Volume fraction of MNP, φ	*((C20(C13))/(C20(C13)+(C21(C14)))*100%	0.212744496				Eq 2
Density of nanofluid, ρnf	ρρp*φ+ ρw*(1-φ)	1665	kg/m³			
Flux of nanofluid,	V*ρnf/Ai	5.63E-02	kg/s/m²	1.63E-01	mol/m²s	
Molar mass of nanoparticles						
Molar mass of core Fe₃O₄		231.54	g/mol			https://www.sigmaaldrich.com/catalog/product/aldrich/637106
Molar mass of octane		114.23	g/mol			
Molar mass of nanofluid		345.77	g/mol	0.34577	kg/mol	
Mass concentration						
Mass concentration znp	fl²/nanofluid	354.17	kg/m³	1024.29	mol/m³	
Diffusion coefficient, Di						
Boltzmann constant, kB		1.38E-23	J/K			
Absolute temperature, T		310.15	K			
Dynamic viscosity of octane, η		5.10E-04	Pa·s			
Radius of nanoparticle, rp		9.5	nm	9.5E-09	m	
Diffusion coefficient, Di	(kBT)/(6πηrp)	4.69E-11	m²/s			
Viscosity of nanofluid						
Viscosity of nanofluid, μnf	ηb/(1-φ)^2.5	9.27E-04	Pa·s			
Heat dissipation, Qmp						
Diameter of NP, DI		19	nm	1.9E-08	m	Miednowski and Sawicki (2013)
Ligand layer thickness, δ		2	nm	2E-09	m	
volume of nanoparticle, vm	(pi*D³*3)/6	3.59069E-24	m³			
Hydrodynamics volume of NP, vh	(pi*(D+2*delta)³)/6	6.36942E-24	m³			
Magnetic field intensity, H0		12	kA/m	12000	A/m	Miednowski and Sawicki (2013)
Frequency of magnetic field, f0		150	kHz	150000	Hz	
Angular frequency, ω	2πf0	942300	Hz	0.001061		
Time of heating, t0		60	min	3600	s	
Product2		3192280000				
Magnetic field, H	H0*cos(omega*t0)	12000	A/m			
Domain magnetization of suspended NP, Md		4.46E+08	A/m			Miednowski and Sawicki (2013)
Saturation magnetization, Ms	Md/Md	4.46E+02	A/m			Miednowski and Sawicki (2013)
ξ2		1.00E-06				
Permeability of free space, μ0	4*pi*1e-7	1.2564E-06	H/m			
Boltzmann constant, kB		1.38E-23	J/K			
Absolute temperature, T0		310.15	K			
Magnetic anisotropy constant, K		4.10E+04	J/m³			Miednowski and Sawicki (2013)
Brownian relaxation time, τb	(3*eta*vh)/(kB*T0)	3.72E-02	s			
Gamma, Γ	(K*vm)/(kB*T0)	3.44E+01				
Neel relaxation time, τN	(sqrt(pi)/2)*tau0*(exp(Gamma))/sqrt(Gamma)	1.00E-09	s			Miednowski and Sawicki (2013)
Relaxation time, τ	(tau*taub)/(tau+taub)	1.00E-05	s			
χ0,ξ	(mu0*Md*H*mu)/(kB*T0)	5.64E-01				
χ'	(mu0*(Md*2)*fl*vm)/(3*kB*T0)	6.99E-01				
χ''	X(*)/(mu)*(coth(xi)-(1/mu))	3.72E-02				
Qnp	μ*mu0*χ*H0*(H0^2)*f0*(omega*tau)/(1+(omega*tau)^2))	3.32E+05	W/m³	See below for all involved models		
Specific heat capacity of nanofluid, cnf						Eq.4a
Specific heat capacity of Octane, chf		2150	J/kg/K			
Specific heat capacity of Fe₃O₄ MNP, cp	Equation 4.16 (specific heat capacity)	765	J/kg/K			Javid et al (2014)
Specific heat capacity of nanofluid, cnf		358.408012	J/kg/K			Eq.3
Thermal conductivity of nanofluid, knf						
Thermal conductivity of Octane, khf		0.137	W/m/K			

Continued

Thermal conductivity of Fe3O4 MNPs	knp	0.5	W/mK
For three dimensional nanoparticle	n	3	
Thermal conductivity of nanofluid, knf	Equation 4.17 (thermal conductivity)	0.18255784	W/mK
The velocity of nanofluid, v			
Velocity of nanofluid at the inlet, v	v=Q/A	3.38E-05	m/s

Supplementary material: Appendix E

In silico study of EPR effect and MFH

Parameters	Formula	Value 1	Units			Value 2	Units	Reference or link		Color code
Density of nanofluid										Input
Volumetric flow rate, $\dot{V}$		3	μL/min			5E-11	m³/s	Javid et al. (2014)		Output
Density MNP, ρ_{np}		5240	kg/m³							Source
Density of base fluid, ρ_f		698.6	kg/m³					https://www.engineeringtoolbox.com/liquids-densities-d_743.html		Equation
Volume fraction of MNP, ϕ	=((C20/C13)/((C20/C13)+(C21/C145)))*100%	0.559118791						Eq 1		
Density of nanofluid, ρ_{nf}	$\rho_{np}\phi+\rho_f(1-\phi)$	3147	kg/m³					Eq 2		
Molar mass of nanoparticles										
Molar mass of core Fe₃O₄		159.687	g/mol							
Molar mass of octane		18.2	g/mol							
Molar mass of nanofluid		177.89	g/mol			0.17789	kg/mol			
Mass concentration										
Mass concentration np	f1*rnanofluid	0.00	kg/m³			0	mol/m³			
Diffusion coefficient, Di										
Boltzmann constant, kB		1.38E-23	J/K							
Absolute temperature, T		310.15	K							
Dynamic viscosity of octane, η		5.10E-04	Pa·s							
Radius of nanoparticles, rp		5	nm			5E-09	m			
Diffusion coefficient, Di	(kBT)/(6πηrp)	8.91E-11	m²/s							
Viscosity of nanofluid										
Viscosity of nanofluid, μnf	ηb(f1-φ)^2.5	3.54E-03	Pa·s							
Heat dissipation, Qnp										
Diameter of NP, Di		10	nm			1E-08	m	Miaskowski and Sawicki (2013)		
Legend layer thickness, δ		2	nm			2E-09	m			
Volume of nanoparticles, vm	(pi*D^3)/6	5.23E-25	m³							
Hydrodynamics volume of NP, Vh	(pi*(D+2*delta)^3)/6	1.436E-24	m³							
Magnetic field Intensity, Hu		12	kA/m			12,000	A/m			
Frequency of magnetic field, ξu		150	kHz			150,000	Hz	Miaskowski and Sawicki (2013)		
Angular frequency, ω	2πf0	942300	Hz			0.00106	ms			a
Time of heating, tu		60	min			3600	s			
Product2	ωt0	3392280000								
Magnetic field, H	H0*cos(omega*t0)	12000	A/m					Miaskowski and Sawicki (2013)		
Domain magnetization of suspended NP, Md		4.46E+08	A/m							
Saturation magnetization, Ms	Ms/Md	4.46E+02	A/m					Miaskowski and Sawicki (2013)		
f2		1.00E-06								
Permeability of free space, μ0	4*pi*1e-7	1.2564E-06	H/m					Miaskowski and Sawicki (2013)		
Boltzmann constant, kB		1.38E-23	J/K							
Absolute temperature, T0		310.15	K							
Magnetic anisotropy constant, K		4.10E+04	J/m³					Miaskowski and Sawicki (2013)		
Brownian relaxation time, τb	(3*πη*Vh)/(kB*T0)	5.01E+00	s			See below for all involved models				
Gamma, Γ	(K*vm)/(kB*T0)	1.00E+00								
Average relaxation time, τ0		1.00E-09	s							
Neel relaxation time, τN	(sqrt(pi)/2)*tau0*(exp(Gamma)/sqrt(Gamma))	1.00E-05	s							
Relaxation time, τ	(tau0*taub)/(tau0+taub)	8.22E+02	s							
χ0, ξ	(mu0*Md*21*H*vm)/(3*kB*T0)	1.02E+01								
χ0	X0*(3/tau)*((coth(ain))-1/(ain))	3.71E-02								
**Qnp	pi*mu0*X0*H0^2*f0*(omega*tau)/(1+(omega*tau)^2)	3.32E+05	W/m³					Eq 16		
Specific heat capacity of nanofluid, cnf										
Specific heat capacity of octane, cbf		2150	J/kg/K					https://www.engineeringtoolbox.com/specific-heat-fluids-d_151.html		
Specific heat capacity of Fe₃O₄ MNP, cp		765	J/kg/K					Javid et al. (2014)		
Specific heat capacity of nanofluid, cnf	$c_{nf} = \frac{\phi \rho_{np} c_p + (1-\phi)\rho_f c_f}{\rho_{np}}$	544.5325483	J/kg/K					Eq 1		

Continued

Thermal conductivity of nanofluid, knf

Property	Symbol	Value	Units	Reference
Thermal conductivity of Octane, kbf	kbf	0.137	W/m·K	https://www.engineeringtoolbox.com/octane-thermal-properties-d_2103.html
Thermal conductivity of Fe₃O₄ MNPs	knp	0.5	W/m·K	Davidi et al. (2016)
For three-dimensional nanoparticle	n	3		
Thermal conductivity of nanofluid, knf	$k_{nf} = k_{bf}\left[\dfrac{k_{np}+(n-1)k_{bf}-(n-1)\phi(k_{bf}-k_{np})}{k_{np}+(n-1)k_{bf}+\phi(k_{bf}-k_{np})}\right]$	0.27606464646	W/m·K	Fig 4

The velocity of nanofluid, v

Property	Formula	Value	Units
Velocity of nanofluids at the inlet, v	v=Q/A	9.93E-01	m/s

The viscosity of nanofluid, eta

Property	Formula	Value	Units
	etabf	5.10E-04	Pa·s
Viscosity of base fluid at the inlet,	etabf/(1-ϕ)^2.5	3.54E-03	Pa·s

$$\phi = \dfrac{\left(\dfrac{m_p}{\rho_p}\right)}{\left(\dfrac{m_p}{\rho_p}+\dfrac{m_{bf}}{\rho_{bf}}\right)} \times 100\%$$

Heat produced by Fe_3O_4 MXPs in the tumor

The power dissipation by MNPs in the presence of external AMF is modeled by the Rosensweig formulation

$$P_{np} = \pi\mu_0 H_0^2 f \chi''$$

where $\mu_0 = 4\pi \times 10^{-7}$ T m/A is the permeability of free space, χ' is the loss component of the magnetic susceptibility χ given by the relation

$$\chi' = \left[\frac{\omega\tau}{1+(\omega\tau)^2}\right]\chi_0 = \left[\frac{2\pi f \tau}{1+(2\pi f \tau)^2}\right]\chi_0$$

where χ_0 is the equilibrium susceptibility assumed to be chord susceptibility corresponding to the Langevin equation

$$L(\xi) = \frac{M}{M_s} = \coth\left(\xi - \frac{1}{\xi}\right)$$

and can be expressed as

$$\chi_0 = \chi_i \frac{3}{\xi}\left[\coth\xi - \frac{1}{\xi}\right], \quad \xi = \frac{\mu_0 M_d H V_M}{k_B T}$$

where χ_i is an initial susceptibility given by

$$\chi_i = \frac{\mu_0 M_d^2 \phi V_M}{3 k_B T}$$

where M_d is domain magnetization, k_B is the Boltzmann constant, and τ is the effective relaxation time given by

$$\frac{1}{\tau} = \frac{1}{\tau_N} + \frac{1}{\tau_B}$$

where τ_N and τ_B are Neel and Brownian relaxation constants, respectively, and are given by

$$\tau_N = \frac{\sqrt{\pi}}{2}\tau_0 \frac{e^\Gamma}{\sqrt{\Gamma}}, \quad \tau_B = \frac{3\eta V_H}{k_B T}$$

where τ_0 being average relaxation time in response to the thermal equilibrium,

$$V_H = \frac{\pi(D+2\delta)^3}{6}$$

and

$$\Gamma = \frac{K V_M}{k_B T}$$

is hydrodynamic volume of MNP,

$$V_M = \frac{\pi D^3}{6}$$

is volume of MNP, η is nanofluid viscosity, K is the magnetocrystalline anisotropy constant, D is the diameter of MNP, and δ is thickness of sorbed surfactant layer. The external applied magnetic field is formulated as

$$H = H_0 \sin(\omega t)$$

where H_0 and f are the amplitude and frequency, respectively, of AMF. The volume fraction of MNPs is defined by

$$\varphi = \frac{M_s}{M_d}$$

where M_s is the saturation magnetization and M_d is the domain magnetization.

Conclusions

A mathematical modeling and simulation approach is applied for newly synthesized core-shell MNPs to treat liver cancer. Hyperthermia processes, infusion, diffusion, temperature distribution, and the fraction of tumor damage are simulated and analyzed quantitatively. The liver tumor is damaged with minimum collateral damage. While comparing constant heat source with variable heat sources, the temperature versus time curves for the three heat sources reveals that the concentration-dependent heat source produces more heat than the remaining heat sources. The core-shell MNPs used in the present study are superior to the preexisting MNPs of the same size for better heat generation. More heat is generated with increasing concentration for a given value of SLP and less SLP is generated with increasing concentration at a fixed value of heat. Moreover, the present study will prove helpful in both preexperimental and postexperimental studies for liver cancer treatment.

Iron oxide MNPs are incorporated to treat a poroelastic brain tumor. The deformation effect is introduced in the hyperthermia process integrated with the thermal effect. The hyperthermia treatment procedure is simulated and analyzed quantitatively. A poroelastic tumor dynamics is solved for deformation displacement, stress, and strain. The nanofluid concentration and temperature are predicted in brain tissue for effective thermal therapy. The brain tumor is damaged with minimum collateral thermal damage. Validation of this study with experimental data further strengthens the present work.

A simulation study is performed using iron oxide MNPs for breast tumor therapies. All the MFH processes are simulated and analyzed quantitatively. The breast tumor is destroyed with minimum collateral thermal damage. The frequency and amplitude of AMF are directly proportional to the elevation of temperature. The finer is the mesh, the more temperature will be increased. This research motivates me to develop a multiscale numerical model to study the transport of nanofluid in the porous tissue. The simulation results show that for dilute nanofluid, the tumor damage largely depends on heating time and MNP distribution in the tumor. While increasing the volume of injected nanofluid causes the MNP concentration to a maximum at the injection site, it has little impact on the penetration depth of nanofluid.

The EPR effect and the nanofluid diffusion in the tumor have been simulated to investigate their behaviors quantitatively for preheating generation planning in hyperthermia treatment of cancer. The velocity of the nanofluid moving through the blood vessel is maximum at the center of the vessel and minimum near the outer walls of the vessel. The velocity of nanofluid at the inlet is larger as compared to the velocity at any other point in the blood vessel. While flowing through the blood vessel, the velocity of the nanofluid in the regions parallel to the epithelial cell spacing in the tumor interstitium is maximum and that in the regions parallel to the edges of the epithelial cells is minimum. The concentration of the nanofluid is the maximum near the blood vessel and it decreases as the nanofluid moves through the tumor interstitium. Both the velocity and concentration of nanofluid from blood vessels to tumor interstitium decrease with time. The mesh-dependent solution for the velocity in the blood vessel reveals that the extremely fine mesh mode produces the best solutions. This work will aid to control the accurate diffusion of nanofluid in porous tumors to produce effective and uniform heating in hyperthermia treatment of cancer. This research will help in planning infusion and diffusion of nanofluid before heat generation in hyperthermia treatment protocols for cancer patients.

Nanofluid around Happel's sphere (HS) in the cell model in cubical and hexagonal packaging is simulated and analyzed quantitatively. The velocity of nanoflow is maximum in the lower and the upper boundaries of the sphere and concentration decreases from inlet to the front boundary of HS and then from back boundary of HS to the outlet. The nanofluid moves through the hexagonal structure with more turbulent flow and with fast speed as compared with the cubical structure. The velocity of nanofluid in cubical structure follows some periodicity, but in a hexagonal structure no such periodicity was observed. Moreover, nanoflow in the hexagonal structure is more deviated than the cubical structure. The concentration is also smoother in cubical structure as compared to the hexagonal package. Moreover, an extremely fine mesh produces better numerical solutions than other mesh modes. One of the recommendations from the current research is that for hexagonal tumor structure, magnetic fluid hyperthermia will be more effective than for cubical structure. The finer the mesh the better will be the solution with a minor addition to the velocity. The velocity and concentration of nanofluid through the porous cubic and hexagonal structures of the porous tumor are also simulated. The simulation results show that the velocity of nanofluid through voids is a maximum and the flow-through of the cubical structure is smoother than the hexagonal structure. The flow is more turbulent and faster in the hexagonal porous structure.

The reacting nanofluid with blood species in porous tissue is investigated through steady-state analysis. The reacting flow is almost homogenous in the porous part of the reactor. Therefore, the velocity at the center is maximum. The concentration c_1 of nanofluid decreases rapidly as its distance increases from the point of injection. This implies that porous tissue is not optimally used. For the concentration of blood species c_2, the reaction is not uniformly distributed in the porous medium and has a maximum close to the radial position of the injecting point.

The MFD generated from the current-carrying coil effectively heat the liver tumor surrounded by the normal tissue. The temperature distribution inside the tumor has been predicted quantitatively. The magnetic vector potential distribution is not the same in all three-coordinate axis direction. The steady-state analysis of temperature distribution is performed and was in good agreement with the analytical solution for cylindrical tissue. The transient analysis of the tumor heating is also performed, and the temperature curve is optimized with experimental data for the best fit. The thermal conductivity of the tumor tissue is estimated for this fitting.

Future work

The underlying research will add more considerations such as the heterogeneous porous tumor structure and correction factors of deposition rates. In future, the research techniques used in this research can be applied to lung, prostate, head, and neck cancers where iron oxide or gold MNPs may be incorporated to produce heat in the tumor. It is predicted that the integration of the numerical study and theoretical modeling will allow a better understanding of MNP transport. We anticipate that current models can be used to help in the future understanding of cancer treatment dynamics with different injected MNPs. This research demands the development of a multiscale computational model to search for MNP transport in porous tissue. This research will continue through the extension of current work by considering the impact of the neighboring micropores, thus dealing with the more realistic phenomenon.

It is interesting to optimize the following parameters: the flow rate of MNPs, maximizing tumor damage, minimizing deposition, heating efficiency, the porosity of the tumor, the elasticity of the tumor, MNP toxicity and shape, surface charge, zeta potential, surface morphology, polydispersity index, the MNP stability and design, hysteresis losses, surface coating, tumor accumulation, anisotropy, space charges and bond bonding, MNP yield, MNP agglomeration, surface stress, etc. In hyperthermia treatments, all these parameters have not been optimized yet. When MNPs move in the immersed flow, all the microforces acting on the particles come into play. So, modeling carrying these microscale effects will also develop new horizons of research in the current field. In the future, it is interesting to investigate the impact of the latest biocompatible MNPs with different sizes, shapes, and morphologies for MFH studies.

When MNPs move near a solid surface suspended in the moving flow, the forces acting on the particles include the van der Waals attractive force, hydrodynamic drag force, electrostatic double-layer force, Brownian motion, lift force, and buoyancy force. The electrostatic double-layer and van der Waals forces act along the normal direction to the surface and are only apparent at the close separation between the particles and the surface. The lift force pushes the particles away from the surface in the direction of motion. When a particle is suspended in a fluid, it experiences the buoyancy force acting in an upward direction. When a particle moves at a high rate, the Besset force acts on it due to turbulent flow conditions.

Besides the drag force, the Magus force can also neglected due to the very small particle size. For submicron-sized particles with a very small relaxation time, the inertia force also vanishes. In the current work, we neglected these microscopic interactions but in the future, we are interested in developing microscale numerical models incorporating these effects, thus dealing with more actual physical phenomena.

Index

Note: Page numbers followed by *f* indicate figures, and *t* indicate tables.

A

Ablation hyperthermia, 5
AMF generated by coil, 99
Analytical and simulated curves, comparison of, 160, 161*f*
Analytical modeling of MFH, 25
Applied magnetic field (AMF), 151
Areola, 95
Arteries, 13

B

BBB. *See* Blood-brain barrier (BBB)
Bioheat equation, 99–100
Biological experiments
  basic types, 1–2
    in silico studies, 2
    in vitro studies, 1–2
    in vivo studies, 2
Biot-Willis's coefficient, 77–78
Blood-brain barrier (BBB), 73–74
Blood vessels, 12–13
  arteries, 13
  capillaries, 13
  veins, 13
Body tissue, modeling transfer of heat in, 48–49
Boltzmann constant, 180–181
Boundary conditions (BCs), 51–52
  Dirichlet boundary condition, 51–52
  Neumann boundary condition, 51
Brain, 73
Brain tumor, 73, 75
  geometry of, 90, 91*f*
  induction heating of, 90, 92*f*
  temperature distribution in, 86–87, 87*f*
Breast, 95
Breast cancer, 95
Breast gland parameters, 98*t*, 118–119, 118*t*
Brinkman model, 139–140
Brownian relaxation, 39–40, 41*f*

C

Cancer
  fundamental types of, 2
  statistics, 2
  traditional techniques used for treat, 2–3, 4*f*
Capillaries, 13
Cerebrum, 73
Chemical species transport node, 99–100, 129
Chemotherapy, 3, 22–23
$CoFe_2O_4$ magnetic nanoparticles, 54–55, 54*f*
  density of, 55
  synthesis of, 8
Compressible and incompressible flow, fluid, 12
Computational analysis of reacting nanofluid
  adding initial condition, boundary conditions, and material, 142–143
  adding physics and geometry construction, 141–142, 142*f*
  mathematical modeling formulation, 139–141
  mesh generation, 144, 144*f*
  properties of nanofluid, 139
  results, 144–148, 145–147*f*, 149*f*
COMSOL multiphysics
  implementation in, 81–82, 81–82*f*
  results and discussions, 82–91
Convection-diffusion equation, 119, 129

D

Darcy's law, 60, 77–78
Degree of tumor injury, 80–81
Diathermia, 5
Diffusion of nanoflow, in tumor interstitium, 118
Diffusion of nanofluid in tumor, 97
Direct needle injection, 10–11
Dirichlet boundary condition, 51–52
Domain magnetization, 180–181
Dynamic light scattering (DLS), 23

E

Effective density, of nanofluid, 50
Enhanced permeation and retention (EPR) effect, 115–116
  diffusion of nanoflow in tumor interstitium, 118
  heat transfer in porous tumor interstitium, 118–119
  nanofluid flow in blood vessel, 117–118

Index

Enhanced permeation and retention (EPR) effect *(Continued)*
  physical properties of nanofluid, 116–117
  results, 119–125
  schematic diagram of, 115–116, 116f

F

Fe_3O_4 magnetic nanoparticles, 75–77
  synthesis
    by facile method, 9
    by Molday method, 8–9
Finite element modeling analysis of breast hyperthermia
  AMF generated by the coil, 99
  mathematical modeling formulation, 96–98
  physical properties of nanofluid, 96
  results, 99–111, 100–111f
  sensitivity analysis, 98
Fluid flow, types of, 11–12
Flux of nanofluid, 50–51
Fraction of tumor necrosis, 98

G

GBM. *See* Glioblastoma multiform (GBM)
Glioblastoma multiform (GBM), 73–74
Gliomas, 73

H

Happel's sphere
  in porous tumor matrix, 129, 130f
  quantitative analysis of velocity of nanofluid, 131, 132f
  simulating nanoflow around mathematical modeling formulation of problem, 128–129
  physical properties of nanofluids, 128
  results, 129–138
  velocity distribution of nanofluid around, 129, 131f

Heat produced by MNPs, in poroelastic brain tissue, 79–80
Heat dissipation
  force acting on nanoparticles, 37
  heating sources used in magnetic fluid hyperthermia, 43–44
  hysteresis curve and coercivity, 39, 40f
  magnetic vector potential, 38
  Maxwell's equations of electromagnetism, 37–38
  by MNPs, 41–43, 56–57, 57t
  Neel and Brownian relaxation, 39–40, 41f
  scalar electric potential, 38–39
Heat generation model parameters, 118–119, 119t
Heating sources, in magnetic fluid hyperthermia, 43–44
Heat in MNPs, 39
Heat produced by Fe_3O_4 MXPs in tumor, 97, 180–181
Heat sources, in concentration and temperature, 58–59
Heat transfer
  in breast tissue, 98
  in porous tumor interstitium, 118–119
Human brain tumor, 74f
Human liver, 54f
Hyperthermia, 4, 74
  for cancer therapy, 5f
  magnetic nanoparticles and, 6–7
  major types of, 4–6
Hysteresis curve and coercivity, 39, 40f

I

Immunotherapy, 3
Infrared radiation heating, 44
Infusion of nanofluid, in tumor, 83, 83f
Initial conditions (ICs), 52
In silico studies, 2
Integrated therapies, 27–28
Interstitial hyperthermia, 6
Intravenous injection, 10
In vitro experimental studies, on MFH, 29

In vitro studies, 1–2
In vivo experimental studies, of MFH, 28–29
In vivo studies, 2
Iron oxide MNPs, 6–7, 7f, 75–77, 76f

L

Laminar and turbulent flow, fluid, 12
Laminar flow, 119, 129
Langevin equation, 180–181
Laser heating, 44
Linear response theory (LRT), 79
Liver, 53
  cancer, 53
  cells, 53
Liver tumor, mathematical modeling, 55–59
  estimation of fraction of tissue necrosis, 57, 58t
  fraction of tumor necrosis, 65, 65f
  heat dissipation by MNPs, 56–57, 57t
  heat sources in concentration and temperature, 58–59, 68, 68f
  mesh generation, 60, 61f
  model validation, 65–67, 66f
  nanofluid diffusion, 56, 62–63, 63f
  nanofluid injection, 55–56, 60
  properties of different MNPs, 67t
  results, 59–69
  simulation of nanoflow from needle tip, 60–62, 61f
  temperature distribution in liver tissue, 63–64, 64f, 67f
  transfer of heat, 57, 58t
Liver tumor tissue, transfer of heat in, 57, 58t
Local hyperthermia, 6
LRT. *See* Linear response theory (LRT)

M

Magnetic field, simulation of, 158–159, 158f
Magnetic fluid hyperthermia (MFH), 53, 151
  analytical modeling of, 25

case study on, 29
with chemotherapy, laser therapy, radiotherapy, or immunotherapy, 27f
heating sources in, 43–44
integrated therapies, 27–28
mathematical modeling approach, 17–25
numerical modeling of, 25–26
optimization in, 26–27
in vitro experimental studies on, 29
in vivo experimental studies of, 28–29
Magnetic flux density (MFD), 152
Magnetic nanoparticles (MNPs), 6–7, 151
and hyperthermia, 6–7
heat dissipation by, 41–43
infiltration of, 10f
loading at tumor site, 10–11
synthesis of, 7–9, 8–9f
Magnetic vector potential, 38
simulation of, 159–160, 159f
Magnetite cationic liposomes (MCLs), 23
Mammary glands, 95
Mathematical modeling
approach toward MFH, 17–25
of cylindrical tumor, 152–157
adding material, initial condition, and boundary conditions, 155–156, 156t
adding physics, studies, and geometry construction, 154–155
magnetic flux density, 152
mesh generation of model, 156–157, 157f, 158t
optimization problem model, 154
steady-state analysis of bioheat transfer, 152–154
transient analytical of bioheat transfer, 154
of enhanced permeation and retention effect
diffusion of nanoflow in tumor interstitium, 118
heat transfer in porous tumor interstitium, 118–119
nanofluid flow in blood vessel, 117–118
physical properties of nanofluid, 116–117
results, 119–125
of liver tumor, 55–59
estimation of fraction of tissue necrosis, 57, 58t
fraction of tumor necrosis, 65, 65f
heat dissipation by MNPs, 56–57, 57t
heat sources in concentration and temperature, 58–59, 68, 68f
mesh generation, 60, 61f
model validation, 65–67, 66f
nanofluid diffusion, 56, 62–63, 63f
nanofluid injection, 55–56, 60
properties of different MNPs, 67t
results, 59–69
simulation of nanoflow from needle tip, 60–62, 61f
temperature distribution in liver tissue, 63–64, 64f, 67f
transfer of heat, 57, 58t
Maxwell's equations of electromagnetism, 37–38
Mesh-dependent analysis, 123–124, 124t
Mesh generation of model, 156–157, 157f, 158t
Microwave heating, 44
$MnFe_2O_4$ MNPs, 54–55, 54f
density of, 55
synthesis of, 8
Modeling estimation of fraction of tumor injury, 49
Modeling nanofluid diffusion, in tumor interstitium, 48
Modeling nanofluid flow, in injecting needle, 47
Modeling nanofluid infusion, in tumor interstitium, 47
Modeling transfer of heat, in body tissue, 48–49
Moderate or mild hyperthermia, 5

N

Nanofluid, 96–97
effective density of, 50
flow in blood vessel, 117–118
flux of, 50–51
mass concentration, 51
physical properties of, 49–50, 116–117
and properties, 151–152
simulation of concentration of, 134–135, 136–137f, 137–138
specific heat capacity, 50
steady-state velocity of, 121–123, 122f
thermal conductivity, 50
viscosity of, 50
volume fraction of, 49
Nanofluid concentration, simulation of, 84–86, 85f
Nanofluid diffusion, in tumor, 56, 62–63, 63f, 128–129
Nanofluid flow, in porous tumor, 128
Nanofluid infusion in tumor, 96–97
Nanofluid injection, in tumor, 55–56, 60
Nanoparticles, force acting on, 37
Nanoscience, 1
Nanotechnology, 1
Navier-Stokes equation, 139–140
Neel and Brownian relaxation constants, 180–181
Neel relaxation, 39–40, 41f
Nelder-Mead optimization in thermal therapy, of cylindrical tumor
materials and methods, 151
mathematical modeling formulation, 152–157
construction of optimization problem model, 154
magnetic flux density, 152
steady-state analysis of bioheat transfer, 152–153
steady-state bioheat transfer model, 153–154
nanofluid and properties, 151–152
results, 158–162
Neumann boundary condition, 51

Index

Nipple, 95
Normal and cancerous female breast, 96f
Numerical modeling, of MFH, 25–26

O

One-, two-, and three-dimensional flow, fluid, 12
Optimization in MFH, 26–27
Optimization problem model, 154
Optimized fitting of simulated curve, 162, 162f

P

Photothermal therapy, 23
Poroelastic brain tissue
    heat produced by MNPs in, 79–80
    heat transfer in, 80
Poroelasticity, simulation of, 83–84, 84f
Poroelastic model, for stress and strain, 84, 85f
Poroelastic tumor
    deformation of, 77–78
    transport of nanofluid in, 78–79
Porosity of tumor, 143
Porous tumor, nanofluid flow in, 128
Primary brain tumor, 73

Q

Quantitative prediction of nanofluid velocity, 135–137, 136f

R

Radiation therapies, 22–23
Radio frequency heating, 44
Radiotherapy, 3, 23
Reacting flow in porous media, 139–140
Regional hyperthermia, 6
Rosensweig formulation, 180–181
Rotational and irrotational flows, fluid, 12

S

Saturation magnetization, 180–181
Scalar electric potential, 38–39
Secondary brain tumor, 73
Simulating nanoflow around Happel's sphere
    mathematical modeling formulation of problem, 128–129
    physical properties of nanofluids, 128
    results, 129–138
Simulation of concentration, of nanofluid, 134–135, 136–137f, 137–138
Simulation of nanofluid concentration, 121–123, 122f
Single-phase flow node, 129
Specific heat capacity, nanofluid, 50
Steady and unsteady flow, fluid, 11
Steady-state analysis, of bioheat transfer in liver tissue, 152–154
Steady-state temperature distribution, simulation of, 160, 160f
Steady-state velocity of nanofluid, 120–121, 122f

T

Temperature-dependent blood perfusion, 87, 88f
Thermal conductivity, of nanofluid, 50
Thermal equilibrium, 180–181
Thermotherapy, 4
Tissue necrosis, estimation of fraction of, 57, 58t
Transient analysis of liver tissue heating, 160–162, 161f
Transport of diluted species, 129
Transport of nanofluid, in poroelastic tumor, 78–79
Tumor
    nanofluid diffusion in, 56
    nanofluid injection in, 55–56
Tumor destruction, 87–89, 88f
Tumor injury
    degree of, 80–81
    modeling estimation of fraction of, 49
Tumor interstitium
    diffusion of nanoflow in, 118
    heat transfer in porous, 118–119
    modeling nanofluid diffusion in, 48
    modeling nanofluid infusion in, 47
    nanofluid diffusion in, 128–129

U

Ultrasound heating, 44
Uniform and nonuniform flow, fluid, 12

V

Veins, 13
Viscosity, of nanofluid, 50
Volume fraction, of nanofluid, 49

W

Whole-body hyperthermia, 6

Printed in the United States
by Baker & Taylor Publisher Services